SEVENTH EDITION

Study Guide to Accompany

Nursing Research

Principles and Methods

DENISE F. POLIT, PhD
President
Humanalysis, Inc.
Saratoga Springs, New York

CHERYL TATANO BECK, DNSc, CNM, FAAN
Professor
University of Connecticut, School of Nursing
Storrs, Connecticut

Visit the Lippincott NursingCenter Website
http://www.nursingcenter.com

Visit the Lippincott Williams & Wilkins Website
http://www.lww.com

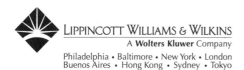
LIPPINCOTT WILLIAMS & WILKINS
A **Wolters Kluwer** Company

Philadelphia • Baltimore • New York • London
Buenos Aires • Hong Kong • Sydney • Tokyo

Ancillary Editor: Doris S. Wray
Compositor: Lippincott Williams & Wilkins
Printer/Binder: RR Donnelley

ISBN: 0-7817-3735-4

9 8 7 6 5 4 3

Preface

This Study Guide has been prepared to complement the seventh edition of Nursing Research: Principles and Methods. The guide provides opportunities to reinforce the acquisition of basic research skills through systematic learning exercises. The book is also intended to help bridge the gap between the passive reading of complex, abstract materials and active participation in the development of research skills through concrete examples and study suggestions.

As in the case of the textbook, this Study Guide was developed on the premise that research examples are a critical component of the learning process. The inclusion of actual and fictitious research examples is designed to instruct (i.e., facilitate the absorption of research concepts); motivate (i.e., encourage curiosity and an interest in acquiring research skills); and stimulate (i.e., suggest topics that might be pursued further by nurse researchers and practicing nurses interested in the utilization of research findings).

The Study Guide consists of 27 chapters—one chapter corresponding to every chapter in the textbook. Each of the 27 chapters (with a few exceptions) consists of five sections:

- *Matching Exercises.* Terms and concepts presented in the textbook are reinforced by having students perform a matching routine that often involves matching the concrete (e.g., actual hypotheses) with the abstract (e.g., type of hypotheses).
- *Completion Exercises.* Sentences are presented in which the student must fill in a missing word or phrase corresponding to important ideas introduced in the textbook.
- *Study Questions.* Each chapter contains two to five short individual exercises relevant to the materials in the textbook, including the preparation of definitions of terms.
- *Application Exercises.* These exercises, geared primarily to the consumers of nursing research, involve opportunities to critique various aspects of a study. Each chapter contains both fictitious research examples and suggestions for one or more actual research examples, which students are asked to evaluate according to a dimension emphasized in the corresponding chapter of the textbook.
- *Special Projects.* This section, geared primarily to the producers of nursing research, offers suggestions for fairly large projects in which, in many cases, an entire classroom could collaborate.

- *Research Reports*. The final section of this Study Guide includes two complete studies for students' critical appraisal.

Like the textbook, this Study Guide is expected to find application at both the undergraduate and graduate levels, and may be of heuristic value to practicing nurses as well.

An appendix provides answers to selected questions in the Study Guide. In addition, the enclosed CD-ROM provides self-study questions that offer further opportunities to reinforce the concepts presented in the textbook.

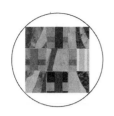

Contents

Additional answers to selected study guide exercises appear in the Instructor's Resource CD-ROM.

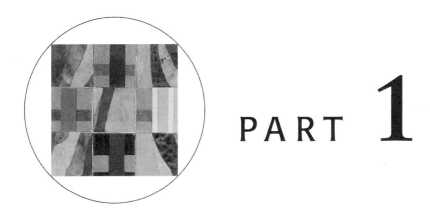

PART 1

Foundations of
Nursing Research

CHAPTER **1**

Introduction to Nursing Research

A. Matching Exercises

1. Match each of the activities in Set B with one of the timeframes in Set A. Indicate the letter corresponding to the appropriate response next to each entry in Set B.

SET A
a. Pre-1970s
b. 1970s and 1980s
c. 1990s to present
d. None of the above

SET B   **RESPONSE**

1. Nursing research focused on nurses themselves   _____

2. Research focus shifted to clinical problems   _____

3. Establishment of the National Institute of Nursing Research
   at the National Institutes of Health   _____

4. Conferences on Research Priorities (CORP) are convened   _____

5. Issue of research utilization becomes more prominent   _____

6. Creation of the professional journal *Nursing Research*   _____

7. Increased interest in outcomes research   _____

8. Goldmark Report is published   _____

9. Greater interest in qualitative research, as evidenced by creation of the journal *Qualitative Health Research*   _____

10. Two professional nursing research journals cease publica-
    tion due to low circulation   _____

2. Match each statement in Set B with one of the paradigms in Set A. Indicate the letter corresponding to the appropriate response next to each entry in Set B.

SET A
a. Positivist paradigm
b. Naturalist paradigm
c. Neither paradigm
d. Both paradigms

SET B	**RESPONSE**
1. Assumes that reality exists and that it can be objectively studied and known	_____
2. Subjectivity in inquiries is considered inevitable and desirable	_____
3. Inquiries rely on external, empirical evidence collected through human senses	_____
4. Deductive processes play an important role	_____
5. Assumes reality is a construction and that many constructions are possible	_____
6. Method of inquiry relies primarily on collecting and analyzing quantitative information	_____
7. Method of inquiry relies primarily on collecting and analyzing narrative, qualitative information	_____
8. Provides a framework for inquiries undertaken by nurse researchers	_____
9. Inquiries give rise to emerging interpretations that are grounded in people's experiences	_____
10. Inquiries are not constrained by ethical issues	_____
11. Has its roots in 19th century philosophers, such as Comte, Mill, Newton, and Locke	_____
12. Inquiries focus on discrete, specific concepts while attempting to control other aspects of a phenomenon	_____

B. Completion Exercises

Write the words or phrases that correctly complete the following sentences.

1. Research in nursing began with _____ .

2. During the early years, most nursing studies focused on _____ .

3. The future direction of nursing research is likely to involve a continuing focus on _____ .

4. The most ingrained source of knowledge, and the one that is the most difficult to challenge, is _____ .

5. The process of developing generalizations from specific observations is referred to as _____ reasoning.

6. The traditional approach to inquiry that uses systematic, controlled procedures is known as the _____ .

7. The paradigm that views reality as multiply constructed is the _____ paradigm.

8. The "scientific method" has as its philosophical underpinnings a school of thought known as _____.

9. Evidence that is rooted in objective reality and gathered through the human senses is known as _____ evidence.

10. The assumption that all phenomena have antecedent causes is called _____ .

11. Because traditional scientific research is not concerned with isolated phenomena, a major goal is _____ beyond those involved in the study.

12. Researchers who reject the classical model of scientific inquiry criticize it for being overly _____.

13. Naturalistic inquiry always takes place in the _____, in naturalistic settings.

14. The type of research that involves the systematic collection and analysis of controlled, numeric information is known as _____.

15. The type of research that involves the systematic collection and analysis of subjective, narrative materials is known as _____.

16. A specific aim of some qualitative research that asks "What is the name of this phenomenon?" is referred to as _____.

C. Study Questions

1. Define the following terms. Compare your definition with the definition in Chapter 1 or in the glossary of the textbook.

   a. Clinical nursing research: _____

   _____

   b. Evidence-based practice: _____

   _____

   c. Producer of nursing research: _____

   _____

   d. Consumer of nursing research: _____

   _____

   e. National Institute of Nursing Research: _____

   _____

   f. Replication: _____

   _____

   g. Evidence hierarchy: _____

   _____

   h. Deductive reasoning: _____

   _____

   i. Inductive reasoning: _____

   _____

   j. Paradigm: _____

   _____

   k. Logical positivism: _____

   _____

   l. Naturalistic paradigm: _____

   _____

   m. Assumption: _____

   _____

    n. Empirical evidence: _____

    _____

    o. Applied research: _____

    _____

    p. Basic research: _____

    _____

2. Why is it important for nurses who will never conduct their own research to understand research methods? _____

    _____

3. What are some potential consequences to the nursing profession if nurses stopped conducting their own research? _____

    _____

4. Students sometimes express concerns about a course in research methods. Complete the following sentences, conveying as honestly as possible your own feelings about research, and discuss your concerns with your class.

    a. I (am/am not) looking forward to this class on nursing research because:

    _____

    b. I think that I would like a course in nursing research methods better if:

    _____

    c. I think that a class in nursing research (will/will not) improve my effectiveness as a nurse because: _____

    _____

5. Below are several research problems. For each, indicate whether you think it is *primarily* an applied or basic research question. Justify your response.

    a. Does movement tempo affect perception of the passage of time?

    _____

    _____

    b. Does follow-up by nurses improve patients' compliance with their medication regimens? _____

    _____

   c. Does the ingestion of cranberry juice reduce urinary tract infections?

     _____

     _____

   d. Is sweat gland activity related to ACTH levels? _____

     _____

   e. Is pain perception associated with a person's level of anxiety? _____

     _____

   f. Does nicotine affect postural muscle tremor?_____

     _____

   g. Does the nurse/patient ratio affect nurses' job satisfaction?_____

     _____

6. Below are descriptions of several research problems. Indicate whether you think the problem is best suited to a qualitative or quantitative approach, and explain your rationale.

   a. What is the decision-making process of AIDS patients seeking treatment? __

     _____

   b. What effect does room temperature have on the colonization rate of bacteria in urinary catheters? _____

     _____

   c. What are sources of stress among nursing home residents? _____

     _____

   d. Does therapeutic touch affect the vital signs of hospitalized patients?_____

     _____

   e. What is the meaning of *hope* among Stage IV cancer patients?_____

     _____

   f. What are the effects of prenatal instruction on the labor and delivery outcomes of pregnant women? _____

     _____

g. What are the health care needs of the homeless, and what barriers do they face in having those needs met?_____

_____

7. What are some of the limitations of quantitative research? What are some of the limitations of qualitative research? Which approach seems best suited to address problems in which you might be interested? Why is that?

_____

_____

_____

D. Application Exercises

Below is a summary of a fictitious study. Read the summary and then respond to the questions that follow.

> Zimmerman (2002) studied the effectiveness of alternative types of messages in encouraging the elderly to come forward for a flu vaccination. All members of a senior citizens' center in a middle-sized community (a total of 500 elderly men and women) were sent a letter advising them that a flu epidemic was anticipated and that the elderly were especially likely to benefit from an immunization. Half the members were sent a letter stressing the benefits of getting a flu shot. The other half were sent a letter stressing the potential dangers of *not* getting a flu shot. To avoid any biases, a lottery-type system was used to determine who got which letter. All the elderly were advised that free immunizations would be available at a community health clinic over a 1-week period and that free transportation would also be made available to them. Zimmerman monitored the rates of coming forward for a flu shot among the two groups of elderly to assess whether one approach of encouragement was more persuasive than the other.

1. Consider the aspects of this study in relation to issues discussed in this chapter. To assist you in your review, here are some guiding questions:

    a. Discuss the relevance of this study to nursing.
    b. Do the methods used in this study suggest that the underlying paradigm is positivism or naturalism? Would it be more appropriate to collect and analyze qualitative or quantitative information? Why do you think this is so?
    c. How would you characterize the purpose of this study? Is its major aim identification, description, exploration, explanation, prediction, or control? Is there more than one purpose?
    d. Would you say this study is an example of basic or applied research?

2. A second brief summary of a fictitious study follows. Read the summary and then respond to questions a to d from Question D.1 in terms of this study.

> Galt (2003) designed a study to explore and describe the meaning of the risk experience among middle-aged men and women whose parents had died of colon cancer and who, therefore, were at elevated risk for colon cancer themselves. A sample of 15 people whose parents had died within the previous 12 months were recruited for the study. In-depth interviews, lasting between 1 and 2 hours, were conducted in sample members' homes. The interviews were tape-recorded and later transcribed. The interviews examined such issues as perceptions of risk, stress associated with risk perceptions, risk-reduction efforts, and coping strategies.

3. Below are several suggested research articles. Skim one or more of these articles and respond to parts a to d of Question D.1 in terms of an actual research study:
   - Gill, S. L. (2001). The little things: Perceptions of breastfeeding support. *Journal of Obstetric, Gynecologic, and Neonatal Nursing, 30,* 401–409.
   - Rossen, E. K., & Knafl, K. A. (2003). Older women's response to residential relocation: Description of transition styles. *Qualitative Health Research, 13,* 20–36.
   - Troy, N. W., & Dalgas-Pelsih, P. (2003). The effectiveness of a self-care intervention for the management of postpartum fatigue. *Applied Nursing Research, 38,* 38–45.
   - Warda, M. R. (2000). Mexican Americans' perceptions of culturally competent care. *Western Journal of Nursing Research, 22,* 203–224.
   - Wikström, B. (2002). Nurses' strategies when providing for patients' aesthetic needs. *Clinical Nursing Research, 11,* 22–33.

E. Special Projects

1. Consider the following research statement:

   The purpose of this study is to determine dyspnea duration and distress among elderly patients presenting for treatment to an emergency department.

The basic purpose of this study as stated is descriptive. Alter the statement in such a way as to design a study whose essential purpose is exploration, explanation, prediction, and control.

2. Think of the last "fact" you learned with respect to clinical nursing practice. Try to discover the ultimate source of this information. Was it tradition ("This is the way it has always been done"), authority ("Dr. So-and-so said so"), logical reasoning ("This has been inferred from previous observations"), or systematic research ("An empirical study discovered this to be the case")?

CHAPTER **2**

Key Concepts and Terms in Qualitative and Quantitative Research

A. Matching Exercises

1. Match each term in Set B with one of the responses in Set A. Indicate the letter corresponding to your response next to each item in Set B.

SET A
a. Term used in quantitative research
b. Term used in qualitative research
c. Term used in both qualitative and quantitative research

SET B	**RESPONSE**
1. Subject	_____
2. Study participant	_____
3. Informant	_____
4. Variable	_____
5. Phenomena	_____
6. Construct	_____
7. Theory	_____
8. Data	_____
9. Bias	_____
10. Credibility	_____
11. Research control	_____
12. Generalizability	_____

2. Match each term in Set B with one (or more) of the terms in Set A. Indicate the letter corresponding to your response next to each item in Set B.

SET A

a. Categorical variable
b. Discrete variable, not categorical
c. Continuous variable
d. Constant

SET B   **RESPONSE**

1. Employment status (working/not working)   _____
2. Dosage of a new drug   _____
3. Pi (π) (to calculate area of a circle)   _____
4. Number of times hospitalized   _____
5. Method of teaching patients (structured versus unstructured)   _____
6. Blood type   _____
7. pH level of urine   _____
8. Pulse rate of a deceased person   _____
9. Membership (versus nonmembership) in a cancer support
   group   _____
10. Birth weight of an infant   _____
11. Presence or absence of decubitus   _____
12. Number of patients in the ICU   _____

3. Match each term in Set B with one of the terms in Set A. Indicate the letter corresponding to your response next to each item in Set B.

SET A

a. Independent variable
b. Dependent variable
c. Either/both

SET B   **RESPONSE**

1. The variable that is the presumed effect   _____
2. The variable that is dichotomous   _____
3. The variable that is the main outcome of interest in the study   _____
4. The variable that is the presumed cause   _____
5. The variable referred to as the criterion variable   _____
6. The variable that is an attribute   _____
7. The variable, "length of stay in hospital"   _____
8. The variable that requires an operational definition   _____

B. Completion Exercises

Write the words or phrases that correctly complete the following sentences.

1. The leader of a team of researchers is known as the _____ or _____.

2. In quantitative studies, the people who are being studied are often referred to as _____; they may be referred to as _____ in both qualitative and quantitative studies.

3. The abstract qualities in which a researcher is interested are referred to by both qualitative and quantitative researchers as _____ _____.

4. A _____, a term used primarily in quantitative research, is a quality of a person, group, setting, or situation that takes on different values.

5. A _____ variable is one that takes on only a few discrete values that have no quantitative meaning.

6. Whereas gender is a categorical variable, height is a(n) _____ variable.

7. The variable presumed to *cause* or influence changes in some other variable is the _____ variable.

8. The variable that the researcher wants to understand, explain, or predict is known as the _____ variable.

9. If a researcher studied the effect of a scheduling assignment on nurses' morale, scheduling assignment would be the _____ variable.

10. A variable that is irrelevant in a quantitative investigation and needs to be controlled is called a(n) _____variable.

11. The pieces of information obtained in the course of a study are collectively known as the _____ .

12. Quantitative researchers carefully specify how to measure concepts of interest, resulting in _____ of those variables.

13. When the data are in the form of narrative descriptions, the data are _____.

14. While quantitative researchers are often interested in studying relationships between variables, qualitative researchers examine _____ _____.

15. "The higher the daily caloric intake, the greater the weight" expresses a presumed _____ relationship.

16. "Men are more likely to suffer depression following the death of their spouses than women" expresses a presumed _____ relationship.

17. Two important criteria for evaluating the quality of quantitative studies are _____ and _____.

18. In qualitative researchers, the worth of the study can be evaluated through assessments of its _____.

19. When researchers use multiple referents to draw conclusions, they are using _____.

20. _____ is an unwanted influence that distorts study results.

21. Contaminating factors need to be controlled in quantitative studies if they are systematically related to both the _____ and the _____.

22. In thinking about how research findings can be used in other settings or contexts, quantitative researchers are concerned about _____ and qualitative researchers are concerned about _____.

C. Study Questions

1. Define the following concepts. Compare your definitions with the definitions in Chapter 2 or in the glossary of the textbook.

   a. Collaborative research: _____

   _____

   b. Informant: _____

   _____

   c. Subject: _____

   _____

d. Construct: _____

_____

e. Variable: _____

_____

f. Heterogeneity: _____

_____

g. Discrete variable: _____

_____

h. Categorical variable: _____

_____

i. Operational definition: _____

_____

j. Data: _____

_____

k. Relationship: _____

_____

l. Cause-and-effect relationship: _____

_____

m. Functional relationship: _____

_____

n. Validity: _____

_____

o. Credibility: _____

_____

p. Triangulation: _____

_____

q. Systematic bias: _____

_____

r. Research control: _____

_____

s. Extraneous variable: _____

_____

t. Mediating variable: _____

_____

u. Transferability:_____

_____

2. Suggest operational definitions for the following concepts.

a. Stress: _____

_____

b. Prematurity of infants: _____

_____

c. Nursing effectiveness: _____

_____

d. Fatigue:_____

_____

e. Pain: _____

_____

f. Obesity: _____

_____

g. Prolonged labor: _____

_____

h. Smoking behavior: _____

_____

i. Cardiac function:_____

_____

j. Respiratory function: _____

_____

3. In each of the following research questions, identify the independent and dependent variables.

a. Does assertiveness training improve the effectiveness of psychiatric nurses?

   Independent: _____

   Dependent: _____

b. Does the postural positioning of patients affect their respiratory function?

   Independent: _____

   Dependent: _____

c. Is the psychological well-being of patients affected by the amount of touch
   received from nursing staff? _____

   Independent: _____

   Dependent: _____

d. Is the incidence of decubitus reduced by more frequent turnings of patients?

   Independent: _____

   Dependent: _____

e. Are people who were abused as children more likely than others to abuse
   their own children? _____

   Independent: _____

   Dependent: _____

f. Is tolerance for pain related to a patient's age and gender? _____

   Independent: _____

   Dependent: _____

g. Are the number of prenatal visits of pregnant women associated with labor
   and delivery outcomes? _____

   Independent: _____

   Dependent: _____

h. Are levels of depression higher among children who experience the death
   of a sibling than among other children? _____

   Independent: _____

   Dependent: _____

i. Is compliance with a medical regimen higher among women than among men? _____

Independent: _____

Dependent: _____

j. Is anxiety in surgical patients affected by structured preoperative teaching?

Independent: _____

Dependent: _____

k. Does participating in a support group enhance coping among family care-givers of AIDS patients? _____

Independent: _____

Dependent: _____

l. Does hearing acuity of the elderly change as a function of the time of day?

Independent: _____

Dependent: _____

m. Is patient satisfaction with nursing care related to the congruity of nurses' and patients' cultural backgrounds? _____

Independent: _____

Dependent: _____

n. Is a woman's educational attainment related to the frequency of breast self-examination? _____

Independent: _____

Dependent: _____

o. Does home birth affect the parents' satisfaction with the childbirth experi-ence? _____

Independent: _____

Dependent: _____

4. Below is a list of variables. For each, think of a research problem for which the variable would be the independent variable, and a second for which it would be the dependent variable. For example, take the variable "birth weight of infants." We might ask, "Does the age of the mother affect the birth weight of her infant?" (dependent variable). Alternatively, our research question might be,

"Does the birth weight of infants (independent variable) affect their sensorimotor development at 6 months of age?" HINT: For the dependent variable problem, ask yourself, "What factors might affect, influence, or cause this variable?" For the independent variable, ask yourself, "What factors does *this* variable influence, cause, or affect?"

a. Body temperature _____

   Independent: _____

   Dependent: _____

b. Amount of sleep _____

   Independent: _____

   Dependent: _____

c. Having versus not having a mammogram _____

   Independent: _____

   Dependent: _____

d. Level of hopefulness in cancer patients _____

   Independent: _____

   Dependent: _____

e. Stress among victims of domestic violence _____

   Independent: _____

   Dependent: _____

D. Application Exercises

1. Below is a summary of a fictitious study. Read the summary and then respond to the questions that follow.

   Savett (2003) observed that different patients react differently to sensory overload in the hospital. He conducted a study to see whether the patients' home environments affect their reactions to hospital noises. Below are the investigator's operational definitions of the research variables.

   Independent Variable: Type of home environment: Based on the patients' self-reports at intake, home environment was defined as the number of household members residing with the patient.

   Dependent Variable: Reaction to hospital noise: Based on responses to five questions (agree/disagree type) answered at discharge, patients were classified as "dissatisfied with noise level" or "not dissatisfied with noise level."

Extraneous Variables
    Age: calculated to the nearest year based on birth date reported at intake
    Gender: patient's gender as recorded on intake form
    Social class: patient's occupation as recorded on intake form

Review and comment on these specifications. Suggest alternatives, and compare the adequacy and completeness of your suggestions with the descriptions provided above. To aid you in this task, here are some guiding questions:

  a. Identify which variables in this study are categorical, discrete, and continuous.
  b. Are the operational definitions of the research variables sufficiently detailed? Do they tell the reader exactly how each variable is to be measured? Can you expand any of the definitions so that they are more precise?
  c. Are the operational definitions good definitions—that is, is there a better way to measure the research variables?
  d. Has the researcher identified reasonable extraneous variables? Are these extraneous variables likely to be related to both the dependent and independent variables? Are there other extraneous variables that the researcher failed to identify but should be controlled? Suggest two or three additional extraneous variables.
  e. What type of relationship is implied by the research question—a functional or causal relationship?
  f. This study is quantitative—Is the question the researcher posed appropriate for a quantitative inquiry? Would a more qualitatively oriented approach have been more appropriate?

2. Below are several suggested research reports for quantitative studies. Read one of them and identify the independent variable(s) and dependent variable(s) of the study. Also, respond to questions a through f from Question D.1 with regard to this actual research study.

  • Hicks, F., & Holm, K. (2003). Self-management desision influences in heart failure. *Clinical Nursing Research, 12,* 69–84.
  • Holditch-Davis, D., Bartlett, T. R., Blickman, A. L., & Miles, M. S. (2003). Posttraumatic stress symptoms in mothers of premature infants. *Journal of Obstetric, Gynecologic, and Neonatal Nursing, 32,* 161–171.
  • Miller, A.M., & Chandler, P.J. (2002). Acculturation, resilience, and depression in midlife women from the former Soviet Union. *Nursing Research, 51,* 26–32.
  • Riedinger, M. S., Dracup, K.A., Brecht, M., Padilla, G., Sarna, L., & Ganz, P. (2001). Quality of life in patients with heart failure: Do gender differences exit? *Heart & Lung, 30,* 105–116.

- Souder, E., & O'Sullivan, P. S. (2000). Nursing documentation versus standardized assessment of cognitive status is hospitalized medical patients. *Applied Nursing Research, 13,* 29–36.

3. A second brief description of a fictitious study follows. Read the description and then respond to the questions that follow.

> Ungar (2002) undertook a study to understand the meaning of compliance with a medical regimen from the patient's perspective among low-income rural patients with a chronic health problem. Ungar noted that although compliance is a widely researched phenomenon, the patient's viewpoint is often ignored. The researcher recruited a sample of 18 men and women ranging in age from 27 to 68 from a health clinic in rural Tennessee. The in-depth interviews, which lasted about 90 minutes on average, were conducted at the clinic. The interviews focused on the nature of the chronic health problem, the nature of the therapeutic regimen, and the meaning of compliance from the informants' perspective.

Review and comment on this study. To aid you in this task, here are some guiding questions.

  a. What is the central phenomenon under study in this research project?
  b. Is the question the researcher posed appropriate for a qualitative inquiry? Would a more quantitatively oriented approach have been more appropriate?
  c. What types of patterns of association, if any, were explored?
  d. What is the setting for the study? Was this setting appropriate?

4. Below are several suggested research articles for qualitative studies. Read one of these articles and respond to parts a to d of Question D.3 in critiquing this actual research study.

- Letvak, S. (2003). The experience of being an older staff nurse. *Western Journal of Nursing Research, 25,* 45–56.
- Lindberg, C. E., & Nolan, L. B. (2001). Women's decision making regarding hyterectomy. *Journal of Obstetrics, Gynecologic, and Neonatal Nursing, 30,* 607–616.
- Nyström, K., & Axelsson, K. (2002). Mothers' experience of being separated from their newborns. *Journal of Obstetrics, Gynecologic, and Neonatal Nursing, 31,* 275–282.
- Volume, C. I. (2000). Hoping to maintain a balance: The concept of hope and the discontinuation of anorexiant medications. *Qualitative Health Research, 10,* 174–187.
- Wilmoth, M. C. (2001). The aftermath of breast cancer: An altered sexual self. *Cancer Nursing, 24,* 278–286.

E. Special Projects

1. Think of five pairs of variables that might have a relationship between them (e.g., smoking status and lung cancer status). For each pair, indicate whether you presume the relationship to be functional or causal. Identify extraneous variables that would need to be controlled when studying those relationships.

2. Suppose you wanted to do a qualitative study of a couple's decision to seek infertility treatment. What types of sites and settings might be appropriate for such a study? How could triangulation be used?

CHAPTER **3**

Overview of the Research Process in Qualitative and Quantitative Studies

A. *Matching Exercises*

1. Match each activity in Set B with one of the options in Set A. Indicate the letter corresponding to your response next to each item in Set B.

SET A
a. An activity in quantitative research
b. An activity in qualitative research
c. An activity in both qualitative and quantitative research
d. An activity in neither quantitative nor qualitative research

SET B   **RESPONSE**

1. Choosing between an experimental or nonexperimental design   _____
2. Ending data collection once saturation has been achieved   _____
3. Developing or evaluating measuring instruments   _____
4. Doing a literature review   _____
5. Seeking financial support for a study   _____
6. Developing a sampling plan that ensures representativeness   _____
7. Gaining entrée into a site and gaining the trust of gate-keepers   _____
8. Taking steps to ensure protection of human rights   _____
9. Developing strategies to avoid data collection   _____

10. Disseminating research results   _____
11. Analyzing the data for major themes   _____
12. Developing hypotheses to be tested statistically   _____

2. Match each activity relating to quantitative studies in Set B with an option in Set A. Indicate the letter corresponding to your response next to each item in Set B.

SET A
a. Conceptual phase
b. Planning phase
c. Empirical phase
d. Analytic phase
e. Dissemination phase

SET B   **RESPONSE**
1. Distributing questionnaires to a group of nursing home residents   _____
2. Deciding which extraneous variables need to be controlled   _____
3. Conducting a literature review   _____
4. Identifying a suitable conceptual framework   _____
5. Deciding to collect data from 300 alcoholics in treatment   _____
6. Determining what percentage of subjects were clinically depressed   _____
7. Presenting a paper at a meeting of the Eastern Nursing Research Society   _____
8. Developing a training session for data collectors   _____
9. Coding data for entry of information onto a computer file   _____
10. Interpreting findings that were contrary to the hypotheses _____

B. Completion Exercises

Write the words or phrases that correctly complete the following sentences.

1. When little is known about a topic or phenomenon, _____ research is likely to be more fruitful than _____ research.

2. In experimental research, researchers introduce a(n)_____, while this is not the case in nonexperimental research.

3. The three research traditions that have been especially fruitful among qualitative nurse researchers include _____, _____, and _____.

4. The research tradition that is concerned with *lived experience* and its meaning is _____.

5. _____ seeks to describe and understand social psychological processes occurring in social settings.

6. There is typically a well-defined, specified set of activities with fairly linear progression in a _____ study.

7. Quantitative researchers may formulate predictions (_____) to be tested during the conceptual phase of the project.

8. If a research problem is clinical in nature, researchers can gain a better appreciation of clinical procedures, clients, and settings by engaging in _____ before designing the study.

9. The overall plan for addressing a question through empirical investigation is called the _____ .

10. The aggregate of people to whom researchers wish to generalize their results is the _____.

11. The actual group of people selected from a larger group to participate in a study is the _____.

12. Typically, the most time-consuming phase of the study is the _____ phase.

13. The task of organizing and synthesizing the information collected in a study is known as _____ .

14. A small-scale trial run of a research study is referred to as a(n) _____.

15. Study findings are communicated in a _____, which is most accessible in the form of a(n)_____.

16. The final phase of a research project is known as the _____ phase.

17. In a qualitative study, an important activity after identifying a research site is developing a strategy for _____ into selected settings within the site.

18. The individuals who control access to research sites or settings are known as the _____.

19. The design of a qualitative study is not predetermined before fieldwork begins, it is a(n) _____ design that responds to information as it is gathered.

20. Quantitative researchers decide in advance how many study participants to include in a study, but qualitative researchers' sampling decisions are often guided by the principle of _____ of the data.

C. Study Questions

1. Define the following concepts. Compare your definition with the definition in Chapter 3 or in the glossary of the textbook.

   a. Experimental research: _____

   _____

   b. Nonexperimental research: _____

   _____

   c. Ethnography: _____

   _____

   d. Literature review: _____

   _____

   e. Clinical fieldwork: _____

   _____

   f. Hypothesis: _____

   _____

   g. Intervention protocol: _____

   _____

   h. Sampling plan: _____

   _____

    i. Data collection plan: _____

          _____

    j. Self-reports: _____

          _____

    k. Pretesting: _____

          _____

    l. Gaining entrée: _____

          _____

   m. Raw data: _____

          _____

    n. Data saturation: _____

          _____

2. Describe what is wrong with the following statements:

    a. Lawton's nonexperimental study focused on the effect of an active variable on two attribute variables.

        _____

        _____

    b. DelSette's experimental study examined the effect of relaxation therapy (the dependent variable) on pain (the independent variable) in cancer patients.

        _____

        _____

    c. Balmuth's grounded theory study of the caregiving process for caretakers of patients with dementia controlled for the extraneous variables of patient age and gender.

        _____

        _____

    d. In Mouzon's phenomenological study of the meaning of futility among AIDS patients, subjects were randomly selected from a list of clinic patients.

        _____

        _____

e. In her experimental study, Izzo determined what types of data would be most appropriate to collect after she got into the field.

_____

_____

3. Read the following report of a phenomenological study and identify segments of *raw data*: Cohen, M. Z., Ley, C., & Tarzian, A. J. (2001). Isolation in blood and marrow transplantation. *Western Journal of Nursing Research, 23,* 592–600. Describe the effect that removal of the raw data would have on the report.

_____

4. Which qualitative research tradition do you think would be most appropriate for the following research questions:

a. How do the health beliefs of Haitian immigrants influence their health-seeking behavior? _____

_____

b. What is it like to be a recovering alcoholic? _____

_____

c. What is the process by which couples adapt to a diagnosis of infertility?

_____

D. Application Exercises

1. Below is a summary of a fictitious quantitative study. Read the summary and then respond to the questions that follow.

Nicolet (2003) conducted a 2-year study to test whether the quality of mother-infant interactions during the first few days postpartum was related to breastfeeding outcome at 8 weeks postpartum. Married women aged 21 to 35 who were in the third trimester of their *first* pregnancies and who had expressed a desire to breastfeed their infants for at least 12 weeks were considered eligible for the study. A sample of 125 pregnant women from Seattle were recruited into the study.

The quality of mother-infant interactions was measured between 48 and 96 hours postpartum in the subjects' homes, using a tool called the Nursing Child Assessment Feeding Scale (NCAFS). The NCAFS consists of six subscales, each of which lists a series of caregiver and/or infant behaviors that Nicolet watched for and recorded during routine feedings. For example, one subscale measures the degree to which the mother fosters her child's social-emotional growth. Scores from the six subscales are summed for a total score that can range from 1 to 76, with higher scores reflecting higher quality interactions. Breastfeeding outcome (breastfeeding one or more times a day versus not breastfeeding at all) was assessed 8 weeks later. Data for the study were collected over a 14-month period.

The findings indicated that women who had continued to breastfeed at 8 weeks postpartum had higher scores on the NCAFS scale than women who had weaned by 8 weeks, consistent with the Nicolet's predictions.

Review and comment on these specifications. Suggest alternatives, and compare the adequacy and completeness of your suggestions with the descriptions provided above. To aid you in this task, here are some guiding questions:

a. Is this study experimental or nonexperimental? If it is experimental, what was the intervention?
b. What extraneous variables, if any, were controlled by the research design? Are there extraneous variables that the researcher failed to identify but that should be controlled? Suggest two or three additional extraneous variables.
c. What was the study population?
d. Which of the three main data collection methods (self-report, observation, biophysiologic measures) was used to collect data?
e. Comment on how long the researcher spent collecting research data.
f. Were hypotheses developed and tested?
g. This study is quantitative. Is the research question appropriate for quantitative inquiry? Would a more qualitatively oriented approach have been more appropriate?

2. Below are several suggested research articles for quantitative studies. Respond to questions a through g from Question D.1 (to the extent possible) with regard to this actual research study.

- Hattan, J., King, L., & Griffiths, P. (2002). The impact of foot massage and guided relaxation following cardiac surgery: A randomized controlled trial. *Journal of Advanced Nursing, 37,* 199–207.
- Morrison-Beedy, D., & Lewis, B. P. (2001). HIV prevention in single, urban women: Condom-use readiness. *Journal of Obstetric, Gynecologic, and Neonatal Nursing, 30,* 148–156.
- Oxley, G. M. (2001). HIV/AIDS knowledge and self-esteem among adolescents. *Clinical Nursing Research, 10,* 214–224.
- Sander Wint, S., Eshelman, D., Steele, J., & Guzzetta, C.E. (2002). Effects of distraction using virtual reality glasses during lumbar punctures in adolescents with cancer. *Oncology Nursing Forum, 29,* E8–E15.
- Sparks, L. (2001). Taking the "ouch" out of injections for children: Using distraction to decrease pain. *MCN, American Journal of Maternal Child Nursing, 26,* 72–78,

3. A second brief description of a fictitious study follows. Read the description and then respond to the questions that follow.

> Ryan (2002) conducted an in-depth study of the experience of caring for an elderly relative. Her focus was on the family members' day-to-day caregiving experience, the stresses to which it gives rise, and the mechanisms the caregivers use to deal with those stresses.
>
> Fifteen primary caregivers of an elderly relative, recruited from the hospital where Ryan worked, participated in the study. All participants were interviewed once in their own homes within 2 weeks after the older relative was discharged from the hospital. Interviews lasted between 2 and 3 hours for each participant. All interviews, which yielded narrative, conversational data, were tape recorded and transcribed. As· Ryan interviewed participants, she realized the importance of gaining the perspective of both male and female caregivers, so she sought additional male participants. Questions for the interviewing evolved from the ongoing analysis of data.
>
> Five major categories of experience were identified. One theme, maintaining routines, is exemplified by the following excerpt:
>
>> I had to begin to arrange my life on a regular schedule or I would not have been able to cope. I get up at 6:30 every morning. I begin to make all the arrangements for the day-I make out a shopping list, get all his medications for the day ready and put them in a pill organizer, organize a little "agenda" for things I think he needs to do. There is so much planning that you have to do. At first, I didn't realize the importance of being well organized. But now that we have a routine, I feel much more in control and much less stressed.

Review and comment on this study. To aid you in this task, here are some guiding questions.

   a. What is the central phenomenon under study in this research project?
   b. Which qualitative research tradition was the basis for this study?
   c. What is the setting for the study? Was this setting appropriate? How difficult do you think it was to gain entrée into this setting?
   d. Which of the three main data collection methods (self-report, observation, biophysiologic measures) was used to collect data?
   e. Comment on the use of raw data in this study.
   f. Is the question the researcher posed appropriate for a qualitative inquiry? Would a more quantitatively oriented approach have been more appropriate?

4. Below are several suggested research articles for qualitative studies. Read one of these articles and respond to parts a to d of Question D.3 in critiquing this actual research study.

   • DeCicco-Bloom, B., & Cohen, D. (2003). Home care nurses: A study of the occurrence of culturally competent care. *Journal of Transcultural Nursing, 14,* 25–31.
   • Dobratz, M.C. (2002). The pattern of the becoming-self in death and dying. *Nursing Science Quarterly, 15,* 137–142.

- Long, T., & Johnson, M. (2001). Living and coping with excessive infantile crying. *Journal of Advanced Nursing, 34,* 155–162.
- Mahoney, J. S. (2001). An ethnographic approach to understanding the illness experience of patients with congestive heart failure and their family members. *Heart & Lung, 30,* 429–436,
- Orshan, S. A., Furniss, K. K., Forst, C., & Santoro, N. (2001). The lived experience of premature ovarian failure. *Journal of Obstetric, Gynecologic, and Neonatal Nursing, 30,* 148–156.

E. Special Projects

1. Suppose you were interested in conducting a quantitative study of the effect of a hysterectomy on women's sexuality and sexual identity. Briefly outline what you might do in the following tasks, as outlined in this chapter:

Step 3 Engage in clinical fieldwork:_____

_____

Step 5 Formulate hypotheses: _____

_____

Step 6 Select a research design: _____

_____

Step 8 Identify the population: _____

_____

Step 9 Develop a sampling plan: _____

_____

Step 10 Specify the methods to measure or operationalize the variables: _____

_____

2. Read one of the studies suggested in Question D.2 and another suggested in D.4. Compare the extent to which you are able to discern the flow of research activities in the two studies.

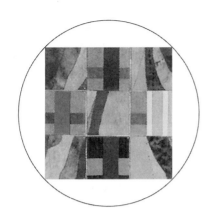

PART 2

Conceptualizing a Research Study

CHAPTER **4**

Research Problems, Research Questions, and Hypotheses

A. Matching Exercises

1. Match each research problem in Set B with one of the statements in Set A. Indicate the letter corresponding to the appropriate response next to each statement in Set B.

SET A
a. Statement of purpose for a qualitative study
b. Statement of purpose for a quantitative study
c. Not a statement of purpose for a research study

SET B	RESPONSE
1. The purpose of this study is to test whether the removal of physical restraints causes behavior changes in elderly patients.	_____
2. The purpose of this project is to facilitate the transition from hospital to home among women who have just given birth.	_____
3. The goal of this project is to explore the process by which an elderly person adjusts to placement in a nursing home.	_____
4. The investigation was designed to document the incidence and prevalence of smoking, alcohol use, and drug use among adolescents aged 12 to 14.	_____
5. The study's purpose was to describe the nature of touch used by parents in touching their preterm infants.	_____

6. The goal is to develop guidelines for spiritually related nursing interventions. _____

7. The purpose of this project is to examine the relationship between race/ethnicity and the use of over-the-counter medications. _____

8. The purpose is to develop an in-depth understanding of patients' feelings of powerlessness in hospital settings. _____

2. Match each of the statements in Set B with one of the terms in Set A. Indicate the letter corresponding to the appropriate response next to each statement in Set B.

SET A
a. Research hypothesis-directional
b. Research hypothesis-nondirectional
c. Null hypothesis
d. Not a hypothesis as stated

SET B   **RESPONSE**

1. First-born infants have higher concentrations of estrogens and progesterone in umbilical cord blood than do later-born infants. _____

2. There is no relationship between participation in prenatal classes and the health outcomes of infants. _____

3. Nursing students are increasingly interested in obtaining advanced degrees. _____

4. Nurse practitioners have more job mobility than do other registered nurses. _____

5. A person's age is related to his or her difficulty in accessing health care. _____

6. Glaucoma can be effectively screened by means of tonometry. _____

7. Increased noise levels result in increased anxiety among hospitalized patients. _____

8. Media exposure regarding the health hazards of smoking is unrelated to the public's smoking habits. _____

9. Patients' compliance with their medication regimens is related to their perceptions of the consequences of non-compliance. _____

10. The primary reason that nurses participate in continuing education programs is for professional advancement.   _____

11. Baccalaureate, diploma, and associate degree nursing graduates differ with respect to technical and clinical skills acquired.   _____

12. A cancer patient's degree of hopefulness regarding the future is unrelated to his or her religiosity.   _____

13. The degree of attachment between infants and their mothers is associated with the infant's status as low birth weight or normal birth weight.   _____

14. The presence of homonymous hemianopia in stroke patients negatively affects their length of stay in hospital.   _____

15. Adjustment to hemodialysis does not vary by the patient's gender.   _____

B. Completion Exercises

Write the words or phrases that correctly complete the following sentences.

1. A(n) _____ is a situation involving an enigmatic, puzzling, or disturbing condition that is of interest to a researcher.

2. A(n) _____ is the specific query the researcher seeks to answer.

3. The accomplishments a researcher hopes to achieve by conducting a study are referred to as the _____ or _____.

4. The five most common sources of ideas for research problems are _____, _____, _____, _____, and _____ .

5. Research questions involving the essence, experience, process, or nature of some phenomenon would likely be addressed in a _____ study.

6. Unavailability of subjects would make a research project _____ .

7. Moral or philosophical questions are inherently _____ .

8. Adequacy of research facilities and time bear on the _____ of the research project.

9. Research hypotheses state a predicted _____ between variables.

10. A hypothesis involves a prediction regarding at least _____ _____ variables.

11. Hypotheses predict the effect of the _____ variable on the _____ variable.

12. A hypothesis that states a prediction regarding two or more independent and two or more dependent variables is called a _____ or _____ hypothesis.

13. The _____ hypothesis states that there is no expected relationship among the research variables.

14. Theories form the basis for _____ hypotheses through the process of _____ .

C. Study Questions

1. Define the following terms. Compare your definition with the definition in Chapter 4 of the textbook or in the glossary of the textbook.

   a. Problem statement: _____

   _____

   b. Statement of purpose: _____

   _____

   c. Research question: _____

   _____

   d. Unresearchable problem: _____

   _____

   e. Unfeasible problem: _____

   _____

f. Hypothesis: _____

_____

g. Inductive hypothesis: _____

_____

h. Deductive hypothesis: _____

_____

i. Simple hypothesis: _____

_____

j. Complex hypothesis: _____

_____

k. Nondirectional hypothesis: _____

_____

l. Null hypothesis: _____

_____

m. Directional hypothesis: _____

_____

2. Each of the following problem statements is either unresearchable or unfeasible as stated. Reword the statements, maintaining the general theme, such that a researchable and feasible problem is developed.

a. What is the best approach for dealing with family members of a dying patient?

REWORDED: _____

b. Should surrogate motherhood be legally prohibited?

REWORDED: _____

c. Should retirement for nurses be mandatory at age 65?

REWORDED: _____

d. Should abortion be available on demand?

REWORDED: _____

e. How can nurses be encouraged to do their own research?

REWORDED: _____

f. What is the best procedure for reducing stress among children before immunization?

REWORDED: _____

g. What role can humor play in improving the well-being of the institutionalized elderly?

REWORDED: _____

3. Below is a list of general topics that could be investigated. Develop a research question for each, making sure that some are questions that could be addressed through qualitative research and that others could be addressed through quantitative research. (HINT: For quantitative research questions, think of these concepts as potential independent or dependent variables; then ask, "What might cause or affect this variable?" and "What might be the consequences or effects of this variable?" This should lead to some ideas for research questions.)

a. Patient comfort _____

_____

b. Psychiatric patients' readmission rates _____

_____

c. Anxiety in hospitalized children _____

_____

d. Elevated blood pressure _____

_____

e. Incidence of sexually transmitted diseases (STDs) _____

_____

f. Patient cooperativeness in the recovery room _____

_____

g. Caregiver stress _____

_____

h. Mother-infant bonding _____

_____

i. Menstrual irregularities _____

_____

4. Below is a list of research questions and statements of purpose. Transform those stated in the interrogative form (as research questions) to the declarative form (as statements of purpose), and vice versa.

   a. Can a nurse counseling program affect sexual readjustment among women after a hysterectomy?

   TRANSFORMED: _____

   b. The purpose of the research is to study the lived experience of parents whose young children have died of cancer.

   TRANSFORMED: _____

   c. What are the consequences of an inadequately maintained sterile environment for tracheal suctioning?

   TRANSFORMED: _____

   d. What are the cues nurses use to determine pain in infants?

   TRANSFORMED: _____

   e. The purpose of the study is to investigate the effect of an AIDS education workshop on teenagers' understanding of AIDS and HIV.

   TRANSFORMED: _____

   f. The purpose of the study is to describe fully patients' responses to transfer from a coronary care unit.

   TRANSFORMED: _____

   g. What effect does the presence of the father in the delivery room have on the mother's satisfaction with the childbirth experience?

   TRANSFORMED: _____

   h. The purpose of the study is to explore why some women fail to perform breast self-examination regularly.

   TRANSFORMED: _____

   i. What is the long-term child-development effect of maternal heroin addiction during pregnancy?

   TRANSFORMED: _____

5. Below are five nondirectional hypotheses. Restate each one as a directional hypothesis.

   a. Tactile stimulation and verbal stimulation yield comparable physiologic arousal among infants with congenital heart disease.

      DIRECTIONAL: _____

   b. Nurses and patients differ in terms of the relative importance they attach to having the patients' physical versus emotional needs met.

      DIRECTIONAL: _____

   c. Type of nursing care (primary versus team) is unrelated to patient satisfaction with the care received.

      DIRECTIONAL: _____

   d. The incidence of decubitus ulcers is related to the frequency of turning patients.

      DIRECTIONAL: _____

   e. Nurses administer the same amount of narcotic analgesics to male and female patients.

      DIRECTIONAL: _____

6. Below are five simple hypotheses. Change each one to a complex hypothesis by adding either a dependent or independent variable.

   a. First-time blood donors experience greater stress during the procedure than donors who have given blood previously.

      COMPLEX HYPOTHESIS: _____

   b. Nurses who initiate more conversation with patients are rated as more effective by patients than those who initiate less conversation.

      COMPLEX HYPOTHESIS: _____

   c. Surgical patients who give high ratings to the informativeness of nursing communications experience less preoperative stress than do patients who give low ratings.

      COMPLEX HYPOTHESIS: _____

   d. Appendectomy patients whose peritoneums are drained with a Penrose drain will experience more peritoneal infection than patients who are not drained.

      COMPLEX HYPOTHESIS: _____

   e. Women who give birth by cesarean delivery are more likely to experience postpartum depression than women who give birth vaginally.

      COMPLEX HYPOTHESIS: _____

7. In Study Questions 5 and 6 above, 10 research hypotheses were provided. Identify the independent and dependent variables in each.

INDEPENDENT VARIABLE(S)	DEPENDENT VARIABLE(S)
5a. _____	_____
5b. _____	_____
5c. _____	_____
5d. _____	_____
5e. _____	_____
6a. _____	_____
6b. _____	_____
6c. _____	_____
6d. _____	_____
6e. _____	_____

8. Below are five statements that are *not* research hypotheses as currently stated. Suggest modifications to these statements that would make them testable research hypotheses.

   a. Relaxation therapy is effective in reducing hypertension.

      HYPOTHESIS: _____

   b. The use of bilingual health care staff produces high utilization rates of health care facilities by ethnic minorities.

      HYPOTHESIS: _____

   c. Nursing students are affected in their choice of clinical specialization by interactions with nursing faculty.

      HYPOTHESIS: _____

   d. Sexually active teenagers have a high rate of using male methods of contraception.

      HYPOTHESIS: _____

   e. In-use intravenous solutions become contaminated within 48 hours.

      HYPOTHESIS: _____

D. Application Exercises

1. Here is a brief description of certain aspects of a fictitious study. Read the description and then respond to the questions that follow.

> Montanari (2003) was interested in studying the notes made by various members of the health care team on patients' hospital charts. She was concerned with several aspects of the chart in terms of its communication potential to various hospital personnel. She began her project with some general questions: Are the nurses' entries on the patient chart used by other staff? Who is most likely to read nurses' entries on the patient chart? Are there particular types of medical conditions that encourage staff utilization of nurses' entries? Do particular types of entries encourage utilization?
>
> Montanari proceeded to reflect on her own experiences and observations relative to these issues and reviewed the literature to find whether other researchers had these problems. Based on her review and reflections, Montanari developed the following hypotheses:

- Nursing notes on patients' charts are referred to infrequently by hospital personnel.
- Physicians refer to nursing notes on the patients' charts less frequently than do other personnel.
- The use of nursing notes by physicians is related to the location of the notes on the chart.
- Nurses perceive that nursing notes are referred to less frequently than they are in fact referred to.
- Nursing notes are more likely to be referred to by hospital personnel if the patient has been hospitalized for more than 5 days than if the patient has been hospitalized for 5 days or fewer.

Review and critique the hypotheses and the process of developing them. Suggest alternative wordings or supplementary hypotheses. To assist you, here are some guiding questions:

   a. Are all the hypotheses testable as stated? What changes (if any) are needed to make all the hypotheses testable?

   b. Are the hypotheses all consistent in format and style? That is, are they directional, nondirectional, or stated in the null form? Suggest changes, if appropriate, that would make them consistent.

   c. Are the hypotheses reasonable (i.e., logical and consistent with your own experience and observations)? Are the hypotheses significant (i.e., do they have the potential to contribute to the nursing profession)?

   d. Based on the general problem the researcher identified, can you generate additional hypotheses that could be tested? Can you suggest modifications to the hypotheses to make them complex rather than simple (i.e., introduce additional independent or dependent variables)?

2. Below are several suggested research articles for studies in which hypotheses were stated. Read the introductory sections of one or more of these articles and identify the research questions and hypotheses. Respond to parts a to d of Question D.1 in terms of these actual research studies.

   - Anderson, R. A., Issel, L. M., & McDaniel, R. R. (2003). Nursing homes as complex adaptive systems. *Nursing Research, 52,* 12–21.
   - DeYoung, S., Just, G., & Harrison, R. (2002). Decreasing aggressive, agitated, or disruptive behavior: perticipation in a behavior management unit. *Journal of Gerontological Nursing, 28,* 22–31.
   - Lee, E. J., McBride-Murry, V., Brody, G., & Parker, V. (2002). Maternal resources, parenting, and dietary patterns among rural African American children in single-parent families. *Public Health Nursing, 19,* 104–111.
   - Nichols, J., & Riegel, B. (2002). The contribution of chronic illness to acceptance of death in hospitalized patients. *Clinical Nursing Research, 11,* 103–115.
   - van Servellen, G., Chang, B., & Lombardi, E. (2002). Acculturation, socioeconomic vulnerability, and quality of life in Spanish-speaking and bilingual Latino HIV-infected men and women. *Western Journal of Nursing Research, 24,* 246–263.

3. Another brief summary of a fictitious study follows. Read the summary and then respond to the questions that follow.

   Zilbermann (2003), herself an asthmatic, noticed that when she experienced dyspnea, she had a tendency to stop moving. A preliminary search of the literature on dyspnea suggested that there was relatively little research on how people with a chronic pulmonary disease react to and cope with the sensation of dyspnea. She conducted a qualitative study guided by the question, how is dyspnea experienced by people with a chronic pulmonary disorder? As she began to discuss this issue with study participants, Zilbermann noticed that people with the three most common types of pulmonary disease—asthma, emphysema, and bronchitis—had developed somewhat different strategies for coping with dyspnea. On the basis of her in-depth interviews (and her observations of several study participants experiencing dyspnea), her final research questions evolved into the following:

   - What are the coping strategies used by patients with different chronic pulmonary diseases to deal with dyspnea?
   - What aspects of the dyspnea experience trigger different coping mechanisms?
   - What are the *patterns* of coping mechanism used by patients (i.e., what strategies are used in what order?)

   Review and critique the researcher's research questions. To assist you, here are some guiding questions.

   a. Comment on the significance of the research questions for the nursing profession.
   b. Does the research question appear to be well suited to a qualitative approach?

    c. Does the researcher's development of her research questions appear to have followed an appropriate process?

    e. Are the research questions worded properly?

4. Below are several suggested research articles. Read the introductory sections of one or more of these articles and identify the research questions. Respond to parts a to d of Question D.3 in terms of these actual research studies.

- Butcher, H. K., Holkup, P. A., Park, M., & Maus, M. (2001). Thematic analysis of the experience of making a decision to place a family member with Alzheimer's disease in a special care unit. *Research in Nursing & Health, 24,* 470–480.
- Callaghan, M. (2003). Nursing morale: What is it like and why? *Journal of Advanced Nursing, 42,* 82–89.
- Canales, M. K., & Bowers, B. J. (2001). Expanding conceptualizations of culturally competent care. *Journal of Advanced Nursing, 36,* 102–111.
- Carter, B. (2002). Chronic pain in childhood and the medical encounter: Professional ventriloquism and hidden voices. *Qualitative Health Research, 12,* 28–41.
- Hines-Martin, V., Malone, M., Kim, S., Brown-Piper, A. (2003) Barriers to mental health care access in an African American population. *Issues in Mental Health Nursing, 24,* 237–256.

E. Special Projects

1. Think of your clinical experience as a student or practicing nurse. Consider some aspect of your work that you particularly enjoy. Is there anything about that part of your work that puzzles, intrigues, or frustrates you? Can you conceive of any procedure, practice, or information that would improve the quality of your work in that area or improve the care you provide? Ask yourself a series of similar questions until a general problem area emerges. Narrow the problem area until you have a workable research problem statement. Assess the problem in terms of the criteria of significance, researchability, feasibility, and interest to you.

2. Below are two sets of variables. Select a variable from each set to generate directional hypotheses. In other words, use one variable in Set A as the independent variable and one variable in Set B as the dependent variable (or vice versa), and make a prediction about the relationship between the two.* Generate five hypotheses in this fashion. Then assess the hypotheses generated in terms of significance, testability, and interest to you.

---

* As one example: Pregnant women who smoke will give birth to babies with lower Apgar scores than women who do not smoke.

SET A
Body temperature
Patients' level of hopefulness
Attitudes toward death
Frequency of medications
Delivery by nurse midwife versus physician
Long-term care residents' quality of life
Patients' self-care
Amount of interaction between nurses and patients' families
Preoperative anxiety levels
Patients' amount of privacy during hospitalization
Smoking status (smokes versus does not smoke)
Recidivism in a psychiatric hospital

SET B
Patient satisfaction with nursing care
Regular versus no exercise
Infant Apgar score
Patients' gender
Effectiveness of nursing care
Patients' capacity for self-care
Patients' compliance with nursing instructions
Amount of analgesics administered
Breastfeeding duration
Nurses' empathy
Patients' pulse rates
Patients' length of stay in hospital

CHAPTER **5**

Reviewing the Literature

A. Matching Exercises

1. Match each statement from Part B with one of the sections in a research report, as listed in Set A. Indicate the letter corresponding to your response next to each of the statements in Set B.

SET A
a. Abstract
b. Introduction
c. Method
d. Results
e. Discussion

SET B   **RESPONSE**

1. Describes the research design   _____

2. In quantitative studies, presents the statistical analyses _____

3. Identifies the research questions or statement of purpose   _____

4. Presents a brief summary of major features of the study   _____

5. Identifies the study sample   _____

6. Offers an interpretation of the study findings   _____

7. In qualitative studies, describes the themes that emerge from the data   _____

8. Offers a rationale for the study and describes its significance   _____

9. Describes how the research data were collected   _____

10. Identifies the study's main limitations   _____

2. Match each of the statements in Set B with one or more of the terms in Set A. Indicate the letter corresponding to the appropriate response next to each entry in Set B.

SET A
a. Electronic databases
b. Print indexes
c. Abstract journals
d. None of the above

SET B   **RESPONSE**

1. Can be accessed only by librarians or information specialists   _____
2. CINAHL   _____
3. Can be searched by subjects/keywords   _____
4. Is an especially efficient means of accessing references   _____
5. Does not include a summary of research studies   _____
6. Are universally available in hospitals and nursing schools   _____
7. Has mapping capabilities   _____
8. MEDLINE   _____
9. Each volume covers a specified time period   _____
10. Manual searches use these   _____

B. Completion Exercises

Write the words or phrases that correctly complete the following sentences.

1. For students who are just beginning to engage in their own research, the most important function of the literature review is likely to be as a source of _____ .

2. The most important type of information to include in a research literature review is _____ .

3. In the context of the research literature, a _____ source is a description of a study written by the researchers who conducted it.

4. For nurses, the most widely used electronic database is _____ _____.

5. Most electronic searches are likely to begin with a _____ search.

6. An electronic search that looks for a topic or keyword as it appears in the text fields of a record is referred to as a _____ search.

7. The two major types of print resources for a bibliographic search are _____ and _____.

8. The type of research reports that students are most likely to read are _____ .

9. The four main sections typically found in research journal articles are: _____, _____, _____, and _____ .

10. Quantity of references is less important in a good literature review than the _____ of the references.

11. The written literature review should paraphrase materials and use a minimum of _____ .

12. The literature review should make clear not only what is known about a problem, but also any _____ in the research.

13. The review should conclude with a _____ of the available evidence.

14. The review should be written in a language of _____, in keeping with the limitations of available methods.

C. Study Questions

1. Define the following terms. Compare your definition with the definition in Chapter 5 or in the glossary of the textbook.

   a. Literature review: _____

   _____

   b. Electronic database: _____

   _____

   c. Mapping: _____

   _____

d. Key word: _____

_____

e. Subject search:_____

_____

f. Textword search: _____

_____

g. Abstract journal: _____

_____

h. Primary source: _____

_____

i. Secondary source:_____

_____

j. Journal article: _____

_____

2. Below are fictitious excerpts from research literature reviews. Each excerpt has a stylistic problem. Change each sentence to make it acceptable stylistically.

a. Most elderly people do not eat a balanced diet.

REVISED: _____

b. Patient characteristics have a significant impact on nursing workload.

REVISED: _____

c. A child's conception of appropriate sick role behavior changes as the child grows older.

REVISED: _____

d. Home birth poses many potential dangers.

REVISED: _____

e. Multiple sclerosis results in considerable anxiety to the family of the patients.

REVISED: _____

f. Studies have proved that most nurses prefer not to work the night shift.

REVISED: _____

g. Life changes are the major cause of stress in adults.

REVISED: _____

h. Stroke rehabilitation programs are most effective when they involve the patients' families.

REVISED: _____

i. It has been proved that psychiatric outpatients have higher than average rates of accidental deaths and suicides.

REVISED: _____

j. The traditional pelvic examination is sufficiently unpleasant to many women that they avoid having the examination.

REVISED: _____

k. It is known that most tonsillectomies performed 3 decades ago were unnecessary.

REVISED: _____

l. Few smokers seriously try to break the smoking habit.

REVISED: _____

m. Severe cutaneous burns often result in hemorrhagic gastric erosions.

REVISED: _____

3. Below are several research questions. Indicate one or more key words that you would use to begin a literature search on this topic.

PROBLEM STATEMENT   **KEY WORDS**

a. How effective are nurse practitioners versus pediatricians with respect to telephone management of acute pediatric illness?   _____

b. Does contingency contracting improve patient compliance with a treatment regimen?   _____

c. What is the decision-making process for a woman considering having an abortion?   _____

d. Is the amount of money a person spends on food related to the adequacy of nutrient intake?   _____

e. Is rehabilitation after spinal cord injury affected by the patient's age and occupation?   _____

   f. What is the course of appetite loss among cancer patients
     undergoing chemotherapy?   _____

   g. What is the effect of alcohol skin preparation before
     insulin injection on the incidence of local and systemic
     infection?   _____

   h. Are bottle-fed babies introduced to solid foods sooner
     than breastfed babies?   _____

   i. Do children raised on vegetarian diets have different
     growth patterns than other children?   _____

4. Read the Keuter et al. (2000) study entitled "Nurses' job satisfaction and organizational climate in a dynamic work environment," which appeared in *Applied
   Nursing Research, 13,* 46–49. Write a summary of the research problem, methods, findings, and conclusions of the study. Your summary should be capable
   of serving as notes for a review of the literature on nurses' job satisfaction in
   relation to organizational climate.

5. Read the following research report (or another article of your choosing).
   Complete as much information as you can about this report using the protocol
   in Figure 5.2 in the textbook:

   Lange, J. W. (2002). Patient identification of caregivers' titles: Do they know
      who you are? *Applied Nursing Research, 15,* 11–18.

D. Application Exercises

1. Below is an excerpt from a fictitious literature review by Edelman (2002) dealing with pelvic inflammatory disease. Read the literature review and then
   respond to the questions that follow.

   There are no universally accepted criteria for defining pelvic inflammatory disease (PID)
   or for categorizing its severity. Furthermore, PID does not exhibit uniformity in its clinical features. Etiologically, cases of acute PID can be divided on the basis of those caused
   by *Neisseria gonorrhoeae,* those caused by nongonococcal bacteria, and those caused by
   a combination of both. Eschenbach and his colleagues (1990) reported that about half of
   the women with PID whom they examined had gonococcal infections. Eschenbach
   (1989) noted that "this difference in etiological agents may explain the clinical differences
   between the gonococcal and nongonococcal PID. The latter may appear less acute and
   may not demonstrate many of the well-defined clinical features associated with gonor-
   rhea" (p. 148). Both gonococcal and nongonococcal PID may result in subsequent
   obstruction of the fallopian tubes, which is among the most common causes of infertility in women. Because fertilized eggs remain in the fallopian tubes for about 3 days, they
   must provide nourishment for the developing zygote. Thus, even a tube that is not completely blocked, but which is severely damaged, can contribute to infertility.

Westrom (1990), in a study of women treated for PID, proved that PID has an impact on subsequent fertility. Records from a sample of 415 women with laparoscopically confirmed PID were reviewed after 9.5 years and compared with those of 100 control subjects who had never been treated for PID. Among the 415 women who had had PID, 88 (21.2%) were involuntarily childless; of these 88, the failure to conceive was due to tubal obstruction in 72 cases (82%). A total of 263 of the 415 subjects (63.4%) had become pregnant. In the control group, only three women (3%) were involuntarily childless.

Westrom's study also revealed a relationship between infertility and the number of PID infections. Tubal occlusion was diagnosed after one infection in 32 women (12.8%); after two infections in 22 cases (35.5%); and after three or more infections in 18 cases (75.0%). Of the 415 women with acute PID in Westrom's sample, 94 (22.7%) experienced more than one infection. Evidence from other studies confirms that a large percentage of women with PID have a history of previous PID and that recurrent PID usually has a nongonococcal etiology (Jacobson & Westrom, 1993; Ringrose, 1994; Eschenbach, 1989).

The number of women affected by PID annually in the United States is unknown and difficult to estimate. According to Rose (1996), Eschenbach and colleagues used data from the National Disease and Therapeutic Index Study and the Hospital Record Study to estimate that over 500,000 cases of PID occurred annually in the United States in the early 1970s. The information from the Hospital Record Study indicated that a mean of over 160,000 patients with PID were hospitalized annually from 1980 through 1983.

Critique this literature review regarding the points made in Chapter 5 of the textbook. To assist you in this task, here are some guiding questions:

a. Is the review well organized? Does the author skip from theme to theme in a disjointed way, or is there a logic to the order of presentation of materials?
b. Is the content of the review appropriate? Did the author use secondary sources when a primary source was available? Are all the references relevant, or does the inclusion of some material appear contrived? Do you have a sense that the author was thorough in uncovering all the relevant materials? Do the references seem outdated? Is there an overdependence on opinion articles and/or anecdotes? Are prior studies merely summarized, or are shortcomings discussed? Does the author indicate what is not known as well as what is?
c. Does the style seem appropriate for a research review? Does the review seem biased or laden with subjective opinions? Is there too little paraphrasing and too much quoting? Does the author use appropriately tentative language in describing the results of earlier studies?

2. Read the literature review section in one of the articles listed below. Critique the review, applying questions a through c from Question D.1.

- Appel, S. J., Harrell, J. S., & Deng, S. (2002). Racial and socioeconomic differences in risk factors for cardiovascular disease among southern rural women. *Nursing Research, 51,* 140–147.

- Desocio, J., Kitzman, H., & Cole, R. (2003). Testing the relationship between self-agency and enactment of health behaviors. *Research in Nursing & Health, 26,* 20–29
- Eliott, J., & Olver, I. (2002). The discursive properties of "hope": A qualitative analysis of cancer patients' speech. *Qualitative Health Research, 12,* 173–193.
- Lawson, M. T. (2002). Nurse practitioner and physician communication styles. *Applied Nursing Research, 15,* 60–66.
- Steward, D. K., & Pridham, K. F. (2002). Growth patterns of extremely low-birth-weight hospitalized preterm infants. *Journal of Obstetric, Gynecologic, and Neonatal Nursing, 31,* 57–65.

3. Below is a brief description of the literature review from a fictitious study by Ward (2002), followed by a critique. Do you agree with the critique? Can you add other comments relevant to issues relating to a literature review, as discussed in Chapter 5 of the textbook?

> **Fictitious Literature Review.** There is now abundant evidence in the medical and epidemiologic literature that pregnant adolescents are at especially high risk of pregnancy complications, of having low-birth-weight infants, and of neonatal deaths (Hillard, 1992; Travis, 1986; Brown, 1989).* Relatively few studies, however, have examined the health status of children born to adolescent mothers after the first few weeks of life. The limited data that are available suggest that children of young mothers continue to be at a disadvantage throughout their infancy and later childhood. For example, Bradley and Lewis (1991) reported that the health of infants born to teenaged African-American mothers was worse than that for infants of older African-American mothers; particular problems were noted with respect to hypoglycemia, respiratory distress syndrome, pneumonia, and seizures. Hughes (1991), in her intensive study of young-parent families, reported an extremely high incidence of health problems among the infants: one fifth had been hospitalized by the time they were 18 months old. According to Tilmon (1989), "These young women are simply not capable of attending to the needs of their children until these problems are so severe they require hospitalization" (p. 315).
>
> Other investigators have proved that accidents and injuries are more prevalent among infants born to teenage mothers. For example, Wright (1990) reported that the risk of infant accidental death was highest among mothers between 15 and 19 years of age. Similarly, Kestecher and Dickinson (1993) found that the most important difference in the health status between 3-year-old children with teenage mothers was the high incidence of injuries and burns to those children with younger mothers.
>
> Few empirical studies have attempted to unravel the factors that might lead to impaired health among the children born to younger mothers. The purpose of this study was to further our understanding of the factors that might lead to greater health problems and less appropriate use of health care among children born to adolescent mothers.
>
> **Critique.** For the most part, Ward appears to have done a fairly good job of organizing and briefly summarizing information about the effect of maternal age on an infant's health status. The research cited appears to be relevant to the research problem, and Ward seems to have relied on primary sources. Without doing a literature review ourselves, it would be difficult to know whether this review is accurate and

* The citations are fictitious.

thorough. We do know, however, that most of the references were fairly old. None of the research cited was conducted in the 3 years preceding publication of Ward's report. It is therefore likely that this review excluded other, more recent research on this topic—research that might have made a difference in Ward's conclusions and formulation of the problem.

Ward's review can also be criticized for being fairly superficial. True, in journal articles, it is common for researchers to be succinct and to cite only the most important relevant studies. It would have been helpful, however, for Ward to make a statement about the believability of the previous research findings based on an assessment of the quality and integrity of the studies.

Two other points about the literature review merit comment. The first is that Ward inappropriately claimed that prior studies "proved" that accidents and injuries are more prevalent among infants of young mothers. The word "proved" should be changed to "found" or some other tentative phrasing. Second, there is an irrelevant and subjective quotation buried in a review that otherwise seems to be objective and neutral. The quote by Tilmon does not belong in this review. At least Ward should have introduced the quote this way: "Findings such as these have led some authorities to speculate about whether young mothers are developmentally prepared to handle the parenting role. For example, Tilmon (1979), who chaired a panel on high-risk infants, made the comment . . . ."

E. Special Projects

1. Read the literature review section from a research article appearing in a nursing journal in the early 1990s (some suggestions follow). Search the literature for more recent research on the topic of the article and update the original researchers' review section. Don't forget to incorporate in your review the findings from the cited research article itself! Here are some possible articles:

   - Bonheur, B., & Young, S.W. (1991). Exercise as a health-promoting lifestyle choice. *Applied Nursing Research, 4,* 2–6.
   - Long, K. A., & Boik, R. J. (1993). Predicting alcohol use in rural children. *Nursing Research, 42,* 79–86.
   - Morse, J. M., & Hutchinson, E. (1991). Releasing restraints: Providing safe care for the elderly. *Research in Nursing & Health, 14,* 382–396.
   - Quinn, M. M. (1991). Attachment between mothers and their Down syndrome infants. *Western Journal of Nursing Research, 13,* 382–396.
   - Singer, N. (1995). Understanding sexual risk behavior from drug users' accounts of their life experiences. *Qualitative Health Research, 5,* 237–249.

2. Select one of the research questions from Question C.3. Conduct a literature search and identify 5 to 10 relevant references. Compare your references with those of your classmates in terms of relevance, recency, and type of information provided.

3. Read one of the studies suggested in Question D.2. Write a two-page summary of the research report, "translating" the information into everyday (i.e., nonresearch) language.

CHAPTER **6**

Developing a Conceptual Context

A. Matching Exercises

1. Match each statement from Set B with one of the phrases in Set A. Indicate the letter corresponding to your response next to each of the statements in Set B.

SET A
a. Classic theory
b. Conceptual framework/model
c. Schematic model
d. Neither a, b, nor c
e. a, b, and c

SET B	**RESPONSE**
1. Makes minimal use of words	_____
2. Uses concepts as building blocks	_____
3. Is essential in the conduct of good research	_____
4. Can be used as a basis for generating hypotheses	_____
5. Can be proved through empirical testing	_____
6. Indicates a system of propositions that assert relationships among variables	_____
7. Consists of interrelated concepts organized in a rational scheme but does not specify formal relationships among the concepts	_____
8. Exists in nature and is awaiting scientific discovery	_____

2. Match each model from Set B with one of the theorists in Set A. Indicate the letter corresponding to your response next to each of the statements in Set B.

SET A
a. Orem
b. Pender
c. Azjen
d. Becker
e. Lazarus-Folkman
f. Mishel

SET B
_____ 1. Theory of Planned Behavior
_____ 2. Health Belief Model
_____ 3. Uncertainty in Illness Theory
_____ 4. Model of Self-Care
_____ 5. Theory of Stress and Coping
_____ 6. Health Promotion Model

B. Completion Exercises

Write the words or phrases that correctly complete the following sentences.

1. Theories are not *found* by scientists, they are _____ .

2. Deductions from theories are referred to as _____ .

3. A _____ is the conceptual underpinnings of a study.

4. Most of the conceptualizations of nursing practice would be called _____ .

5. Schematic models attempt to represent reality with a minimal use of _____ .

6. A statistical model predicts the _____ that a certain behavior or characteristic will exist, given the occurrence of other phenomena.

7. In the statistical model $Y = \beta_1 X_1 + \beta_2 X_2 + e$, the βs are _____ .

8. The four central concepts of conceptual models in nursing are _____, _____ , _____, and _____ .

9. The basic intellectual process underlying theory development is _____ .

10. The acronym HBM stands for the _____ .

11. Theoretical frameworks from non-nursing disciplines are sometimes referred to as _____ .

12. Qualitative researchers sometimes seek to develop a _____ theory, a conceptualization of a phenomenon rooted in the researcher's observations.

C. Study Questions

1. Define the following terms. Compare your definition with the definition in Chapter 6 or in the glossary of the textbook.

   a. Descriptive theory: _____

   _____

   b. Macrotheory: _____

   _____

   c. Middle-range theory: _____

   _____

   d. Laws:_____

   _____

   e. Conceptual framework: _____

   _____

   f. Conceptual definition: _____

   _____

   g. Schematic model: _____

   _____

   h. Statistical model: _____

   _____

2. Read some recent issues of a nursing research journal. Identify at least three different theories cited by nurse researchers in these research reports.

3. Using the statistical model presented in Chapter 6 of the textbook, suggest an alternative example for the Y (the dependent variable) and Xs the (independent variables). That is, hypothesize that some behavior or outcome of interest (Y) is due to the combined influence of four other factors (Xs).

4. Choose one of the conceptual frameworks of nursing that were described in this chapter. Develop a research hypothesis based on this framework.

D. Application Exercises

1. Below is a description of the conceptual framework for a fictitious study. Read the summary and then respond to the questions that follow.

> Wilcox (2003) developed a study derived from Rotter's social learning theory. Social learning theory postulates that human behaviors are contingent on the individual's expectancy that a particular behavior will be reinforced (rewarded). A key concept is locus of control, which is conceptualized as the degree to which a person perceives that rewards are a function of his or her own actions as opposed to external forces. Internal controllers are those who perceive themselves and their behavior as the major determinants of the reinforcement, while external controllers are those who tend to see little, if any, relationship between their own actions and subsequent reinforcement.
>
> Wilcox hypothesized that people with an internal locus-of-control orientation would be more likely to engage in preventive health care activities than those with an external orientation. As a rationale for this hypothesis, she reasoned that "internal" people see themselves as capable of controlling health outcomes, while externally oriented people see forces outside of their control as the major determinants of health outcomes; the "externals" are, therefore, less likely to engage in preventive health care behaviors. To test her hypothesis, Wilcox operationalized "willingness to engage in preventive health care activities" as enrollment in a health maintenance organization (HMO) among a group of employees who were offered a choice between a traditional medical benefits package and HMO membership. Five hundred employees hired by a large industrial firm were administered a test that measured locus of control as part of the application process. Each new employee was offered a choice between the two medical programs. The 187 employees who chose HMO membership were found to have significantly higher (i.e., more internal) scores on the locus-of-control measure than the 313 employees who elected the traditional medical plan, thereby supporting Wilcox's hypothesis.

Review and critique the above study, particularly with respect to its theoretical basis. To assist you in your critique, here are some guiding questions:

a. Examine the study variables. To what extent are they congruent with the conceptual perspective of the study's theoretical framework? Can you offer any suggestions for a different theoretical basis than the one used?

b. Do the hypotheses and research methods flow naturally from the theoretical framework, or does the link between them seem contrived?

c. In what way, if any, did the use of a theory enhance the value of this study? Compare the meaningfulness of the study as described with what it would have been had the same hypothesis been tested in the absence of a theory.

d. In what way, if any, did the outcome of the study affect the value of the theory? If the outcome had been different (e.g., no differences, or differences opposite to those predicted), what effect would that have had on the theory?

2. Read the introductory sections of one of the actual research studies cited below. Apply questions a through d from Question D.1 to one of these studies.

   - Blue, C. L., & Valley, J. M. (2002). Predictors of influenza vaccine: Acceptance among healthy adult workers. *AAOHN Journal, 50,* 227–233.
   - Boonpongmanee, C., Zauszniewski, J. A., & Morris, D. L. (2003). Resourcefulness and self-care in pregnant women with HIV. *Western Journal of Nursing Research, 25,* 75–92
   - Doran, D. I., Sidani, S., Keatings, M., & Doidge, D. (2002). An empirical test of the Nursing Role Effectiveness Model. *Journal of Advanced Nursing, 38,* 29–39.
   - Reynaud, S. N., & Meeker, B. J. (2002). Coping style of older adults with ostomies, *Journal of Gerontological Nursing, 28,* 30–36.
   - Valois, P., Turgeon. H., Godin, G., Blondeau, D., & Cote, F. (2001) Influence of a persuasive strategy on nursing students' beliefs and attitudes toward provision of care to people living with HIV/AIDS. *Journal of Nursing Education, 40,* 354–358.
   - Wang, H. H. (2001). A comparison of two models of life-promoting lifestyle in rural elderly Taiwanese women. *Public Health Nursing, 18,* 204–211.

3. Brunelle (2002) conducted a study to examine factors related to the health and health care of children born to adolescent mothers. Below is a brief description of the conceptual framework used in this fictitious study, followed by a critique. Do you agree with the critique? Can you add other comments relevant to issues relating to the conceptual framework, as discussed in Chapter 6 of the textbook?

   Fictitious conceptual framework. There is now abundant evidence in the medical and epidemiologic literature that adolescents are at especially high risk of pregnancy complications and that their infants have a higher-than-average rate of low-birth-weight and neonatal death. Relatively few studies, however, have examined the health status of children born to adolescent mothers after the first few weeks of life. The limited data that are available suggest that children of young mothers continue to be at a disadvantage throughout their infancy and later childhood. The purpose of this study was to further our understanding of the factors that might lead to greater health problems and less appropriate use of health care among children born to adolescent mothers.

   The theoretical framework for this study was the Health Belief Model (HBM). This model postulates that health-seeking behavior is influenced by the perceived threat posed by a health problem and the perceived value of actions designed to reduce the threat (Becker, 1978). Within the HBM, perceived susceptibility refers to a person's perception that a health problem is personally relevant. It is hypothesized that young mothers are developmentally unable to perceive their own (or their infant's) susceptibility to health risk accurately. Furthermore, adolescent mothers are hypothesized to be less likely, because of their developmental immaturity, to perceive accurately the severity of their infants' health problems and less likely to assess accurately the benefit of appropriate interventions than older mothers. Finally, teenaged mothers are expected to evaluate less accurately the costs (which, in the HBM, include the complexity, duration, accessibility, and financial costs) of securing treatment. In summary, the HBM provides an excellent vehicle for testing the mechanisms through which children of young mothers are at higher-than-average risk of severe health problems and are less likely to receive appropriate health care.

Critique. The theoretical basis for Brunelle's study was a non-nursing model that has frequently been applied to problems relating to health care use. This model appears to have provided an appropriate conceptual basis for the study. Although Brunelle might have provided somewhat more information regarding features of the HBM, she did explain the HBM sufficiently to clarify the basis for her hypotheses. Her hypotheses are clearly linked to the model and appear to be logically related to the problem at hand.

Previous research had yielded descriptive information suggesting that children born to teenage mothers are at higher risk than other children for health problems and inadequate health care. By basing this research on the HBM, Brunelle was attempting to explain why this might be so. She hypothesized that the differences between the children of older and younger mothers reflect the younger mothers' appraisals of their children's needs and of the value of obtaining treatment. By operationalizing the key concepts in the HBM (e.g., perceived susceptibility, perceived severity of the illness, perceived cost of securing treatment), Brunelle's hypotheses can be put to an empirical test. If Brunelle found differences between older and young mothers in their appraisals of their children's health care needs, progress would have been made toward explaining differences in the children's health outcomes. If, however, Brunelle found no differences in mothers' appraisals, another researcher interested in the same problem would have to evaluate whether a different conceptual framework might be more productive in helping to explain differences in children's health and health care, or whether Brunelle failed—through her research design decisions—to test the HBM adequately.

E. Special Projects

1. One proposition of reinforcement theory is that *if* a behavior is rewarded (reinforced), *then* the behavior will be repeated (learned). Based on this theory and on your observation of behaviors in health settings or schools of nursing, suggest three nursing research problem statements.

2. Select one of the research questions in Exercise C.4., Chapter 3, of this study guide (or identify a research question of your own). Abstract a generalized issue (or several issues) from the statement. Search for an existing theory that might be applicable and appropriate.

3. Develop a researchable problem statement based on Orem's Model of Self-Care or Pender's Health Promotion Model (Figure 6-1 in the textbook).

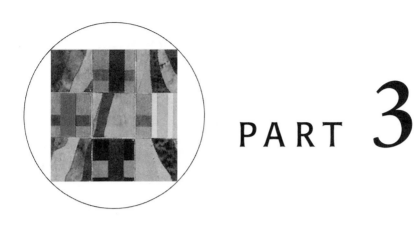

PART 3

Designs for Nursing Research

CHAPTER **7**

Designing Ethical Research

A. *Matching Exercises*

Match each description in Set B with one of the procedures used to protect human subjects listed in Set A. Indicate the letter corresponding to the appropriate response next to each entry in Set B.

SET A
a. Freedom from harm or exploitation
b. Informed consent
c. Anonymity
d. Confidentiality

SET B   **RESPONSE**

1. A questionnaire distributed by mail bears an identification number in one corner. Respondents are assured their responses will not be individually divulged. _____

2. Hospitalized children included in a study, and their parents, are told the study's aims and procedures. Parents are asked to sign an authorization. _____

3. Respondents in a study in which the same respondents will participate twice by completing questionnaires are asked to place their own four-digit identification number on the questionnaire and to memorize the number. Respondents are assured their answers will remain private. _____

4. Study participants in an in-depth study of family members' coping with a natural disaster renegotiate the terms of their participation at successive interviews. _____

5. Women who recently had a mastectomy are studied in terms of psychological consequences. In the interview, sensitive questions are carefully worded. After the interview, debriefing with the respondent determines the need for psychological support.   _____

6. Women interviewed in the above study (question 5) are told that the information they provide will not be individually divulged.   _____

7. Subjects who volunteered for an experimental treatment for AIDS are warned of potential side effects and are asked to sign a waiver.   _____

8. After determining that a new intervention resulted in subject discomfort, the researcher discontinued the study.   _____

9. Unmarked questionnaires are distributed to a class of nursing students. The instructions indicate that responses will not be individually divulged.   _____

10. The researcher assures subjects that they will be interviewed as part of the study at a single point in time and adheres to this promise.   _____

11. A questionnaire distributed to a sample of nursing students includes a statement indicating that completion and submission of the questionnaire will be construed as voluntary participation in a study.   _____

12. The names, ages, and occupations of study participants whose interviews are excerpted in the research report are not divulged.   _____

B. COMPLETION EXERCISES

Write the words or phrases that correctly complete the following sentences.

1. Ethical _____ arise when participants' rights and the demands of science are put in direct conflict.

2. One of the first internationally recognized efforts to establish ethical standards was the _____ .

3. In the U. S., the National Commission for the Protection of Human Subjects of Biomedical and Behavioral Research issued a well-known set of guidelines known as the _____.

4. The most straightforward ethical precept is the protection of subjects from

   _____ .

5. Risks that are no greater than those ordinarily encountered in daily life are

   referred to as _____ .

6. The right to _____ means that prospective subjects have the

   right to voluntarily decide whether to participate in a study, without risk of

   penalty.

7. Researchers adhere to the principle of _____ by fully

   describing to participants the nature of the study and the likely risks and ben-

   efits of participation.

8. When researchers cannot link research information to the people who provid-

   ed it, the condition known as _____ has prevailed.

9. Special procedures are often required to safeguard the rights of _____

   subjects.

10. Committees established in institutions to review proposed research procedures

    with respect to their adherence to ethical guidelines are often called IRBs, or

    _____ .

C. Study Questions

1. Define the following terms. Compare your definition with the definition in
   Chapter 7 or in the glossary of the textbook.

   a. Code of ethics: _____

   _____

   b. Beneficence: _____

   _____

   c. Debriefing: _____

   _____

   d. Stipends: _____

   _____

e. Risk/benefit ratio: _____

_____

f. Process consent: _____

_____

g. Coercion: _____

_____

h. Covert data collection: _____

_____

i. Deception: _____

_____

j. Confidentiality: _____

_____

k. Informed consent: _____

_____

l. Expedited review: _____

_____

m. Vulnerable subjects: _____

_____

n. Implied consent: _____

_____

2. Below are descriptions of several research studies. Suggest some ethical dilemmas that are likely to emerge for each.

a. A study of coping behaviors among rape victims _____

_____

_____

b. An unobtrusive observational study of fathers' behaviors in the delivery room _____

_____

_____

c. An interview study of the determinants of heroin addiction _____

_____

_____

d. A study of dependence among mentally retarded children _____

_____

_____

e. An investigation of the verbal interactions among schizophrenic patients __

_____

_____

f. A study of the effects of a new drug on humans _____

_____

_____

3. The following two studies involved the use of vulnerable subjects. Evaluate the ethical aspects of one or both of these studies, paying special attention to the manner in which the subjects' heightened vulnerability was handled.

   - Shyu, Y. L. (2002). A conceptual framework for understanding the process of family caregiving to frail elders in Taiwan. *Research in Nursing & Health, 25,* 111–121.
   - Wise, B. V. (2002). In their own words: The lived experience of pediatric liver transplantation. *Qualitative Health Research, 12,* 74–90.

4. In the textbook, two unethical studies were described (the study of syphilis among African-American men and the study in which live cancer cells were injected in elderly patients). Identify which ethical principles were transgressed in these studies.

5. A stipend of $15 was paid to the women who completed a questionnaire concerning their sexual histories and other topics in the following study:

   Kenney, J. W., Reinholtz, C., & Angelini, P. J. (1998). Sexual abuse, sex before age 16, and high-risk behaviors of your females with sexually transmitted disease. *Journal of Obstetric, Gynecologic, and Neonatal Nursing, 27,* 54–63.

   Read the introductory sections of the report, and comment on the appropriateness of the stipend.

D. Application Exercises

1. Here is a brief description of ethical aspects of a fictitious study. Read the description and then respond to the questions that follow.

Singleton (2003) investigated the behaviors of nursing students in crisis or emergency situations. She was interested in comparing the behaviors of students from baccalaureate versus diploma programs to determine the adequacy of the preparation given to students in handling emergencies. Fifty students from both types of programs volunteered to participate in the study. The investigator wanted to observe reactions to crises as they might occur naturally, so participants were not told the exact nature of the study. Each student was instructed to take the vital signs of a "patient," purportedly to evaluate the students' skills. The "patient," who was described as another student but who in fact was a confederate of the investigator, simulated an epileptic seizure while the vital signs were being taken. A research assistant, who was unaware of the purpose of the study and who did not know the educational background of the subjects, observed the timeliness and appropriateness of the students' responses to the situation through a one-way mirror. Participants were not required to fill out any forms that recorded their identities. Immediately after participation, the students were debriefed as to the true nature of the study and were paid a $10 stipend.

Consider the aspects of this study in terms of the issues discussed in this chapter. To assist you in your review, here are some guiding questions:

  a. Were the study participants in this study at risk of physical or psychological harm? Were they at risk of exploitation?
  b. Did participants derive any benefits from taking part in the study? Did the nursing community or society at large benefit? How would you assess the risk/benefit ratio?
  c. Were the participants' rights to self-determination violated? Was there any coercion involved? Was full disclosure made before participation? Was informed consent given to participants and documented?
  d. Were participants treated fairly? Was their right to privacy protected?
  e. What ethical dilemmas does this study present? How, if at all, can the dilemmas be resolved? To what extent *were* they resolved?
  f. What type of human subjects review would be appropriate for a study such as the one described?

2. Read one or more of the articles listed below. Respond to questions a through f from Question D.1 in terms of these actual research studies.

  • Hodges, H. F., Keeley, A. C., & Grier, E. C. (2001) Masterworks of art and chronic illness experiences in the elderly. *Journal of Advanced Nursing, 36,* 389–398.
  • Johansson, E., & Winkvist, A. (2002). Trust and transparency in human encounters in tuberculosis control: Lessons learned from Vietnam. *Qualitative Health Research, 12,* 473–491.

- Pender, N. J., Bar-Or, O., Wilk, B., & Mitchell, S. (2002). Self-efficacy and perceived exertion of girls during exercise. *Nursing Research, 51,* 86–92.
- Stewart, J. L. (2003). "Getting used to it": children finding the ordinary and routine in the uncertain context of cancer. *Qualitative Health Research, 13,* 394–407.
- Swallow, V. M., & Jacoby A. (2001). Mothers' coping in chronic childhood illness: The effect of presymptomatic diagnosis of vesicoureteric reflux. *Journal of Advanced Nursing, 33,* 69–78.

3. Below is a brief description of the ethical aspects of a fictitious study, followed by a critique. Do you agree with the critique? Can you add other comments relevant to the ethical dimensions of the study?

Fictitious Study. Fortune (2002) conducted an in-depth study of nursing home patients to determine if their perceptions about personal control over decision making differed from the perceptions of the nursing staff. The investigator studied 25 nurse-patient dyads to determine whether there were differing perceptions and experiences regarding control over activities of daily living, such as arising, eating, and dressing. All of the nurses in the study were employed by the nursing home in which the patients resided. Because the nursing home had no IRB, Fortune sought permission to conduct the study from the nursing home administrator. She also obtained the consent of the legal guardian or responsible family member of each patient. All study participants were fully informed about the nature of the study. The researcher assured the nurses and the legal guardians and family members of the patients of the confidentiality of the information and obtained their consent in writing. Data were gathered primarily through in-depth interviews with the patients and the nurses, at separate times. The researcher also observed interactions between the patients and nurses. The findings from the study showed that patients perceived that they had more control over all aspects of the activities of daily living (except eating) than the nurses perceived that they had. Excerpts from the interviews were used verbatim in the research report, but Fortune did not divulge the location of the nursing home, and she used fictitious names for all participants.

Critique. Fortune did a reasonably good job of adhering to basic ethical principles in the conduct of her research. She obtained written permission to conduct the study from the nursing home administrator, and she obtained informed consent from the nurse participants and the legal guardians or family members of the patients. The study participants were not put at risk in any way, and the patients who participated may actually have enjoyed the opportunity to have a conversation with the researcher. Fortune also took appropriate steps to maintain the confidentiality of participants. It is still unclear, however, whether the patients knowingly and willingly participated in the research. Nursing home residents are a vulnerable group. They may not have been aware of their right to refuse to be interviewed without fear of repercussion. Fortune could have enhanced the ethical aspects of the study by taking more vigorous steps to obtain the informed, voluntary consent of the nursing home residents or to exclude patients who could not reasonably be expected to understand the researcher's request. Given the vulnerability of the group, Fortune might also have established her own review panel composed of peers and interested lay people to review the ethical dimensions of her project. Debriefing sessions with study participants would also have been appropriate.

E. Special Projects

1. Prepare. a brief summary of a hypothetical study in which there are at least three major benefits to people participating in the study.

2. Prepare a brief summary of a hypothetical study in which the costs and benefits are both high. When the costs and benefits are essentially balanced, how should the researcher decide whether or not to proceed?

3. Skim the following research report, and draft an informed consent form for this study:

   Carruth, A. K., Skarke, L., Moffett, B., & Prestholdt, C. (2002). Nonfatal injury experiences among women on family farms. *Clinical Nursing Research, 11,* 130–148.

CHAPTER **8**

Designing Quantitative Studies

A. *Matching Exercises*

1. Match each research question from Set B with a phrase from Set A that indicates the nature of the comparison implied in the research question. Indicate the letter corresponding to your response next to each statement in Set B.

SET A
a. Comparison of two or more groups
b. Comparison of a group at two or more points in time
c. Comparison of a group under different circumstances
d. Comparison of relative rankings

SET B   **RESPONSE**

1. Is morale among the institutionalized elderly related to their self-care abilities? _____

2. Do married and unmarried pregnant women differ in their perceptions of nursing care after delivery? _____

3. Do women instructed in the benefits of breast self-examination (BSE) increase the frequency of BSE? _____

4. Do men and women have different styles of coping after a spouse's death? _____

5. Do patients give different oral temperature readings immediately after they have ingested iced water compared with when no iced water is ingested? _____

6. Is hospital noise intensity related to patients' amount of time spent in rapid-eye movement (REM) sleep? _____

7. Are women who run regularly more likely than nonrunners to develop amenorrhea?   _____

8. Does the level of maternal attachment among pregnant women change after they have seen a sonogram image of their fetus?   _____

9. Are there fewer complaints from patients on days when they are fed breakfast at 8:00 AM than on days when they are fed breakfast at 7:00 AM?   _____

10. Are there differences in the levels of depression among U.S. immigrants from Central America, Asia, and Europe?   _____

2. Match each design representation from Set B with one of the design types from Set A. Indicate the letter corresponding to your response next to each item in Set B.

SET A
a. True experimental design
b. Quasi-experimental design
c. Preexperimental design
d. Nonexperimental design

SET B   **RESPONSE**

1. $\dfrac{\quad X \quad O}{O}$ _____

2. $O_1 O_2 O_3 O_4 \quad X \quad O_5 O_6 O_7 O_8$ _____

3. $\dfrac{R \quad X \quad O}{R \qquad\quad O}$ _____

4. $\dfrac{O_1 \quad X \quad O_2}{O_1 \qquad\quad O_2}$ _____

5. $O_1 \quad X \quad O_2$ _____

6. $\dfrac{\begin{array}{ccc} R & X_1 & O \\ R & X_2 & O \\ R & & O \end{array}}{}$ _____

7. $\dfrac{O_1 \qquad\qquad O_2}{O_1 \qquad\qquad O_2}$ _____

8. $\dfrac{O_1 O_2 O_3 O_4 \quad X \quad O_5 O_6 O_7 O_8}{O_1 O_2 O_3 O_4 \qquad\quad O_5 O_6 O_7 O_8}$ _____

3. Match each problem statement from Set B with one (or more) of the phrases from Set A that indicates a potential reason for using a nonexperimental

approach. Indicate the letter(s) corresponding to your response next to each statement in Set B.

SET A
a. Independent variable cannot be manipulated
b. Ethical constraints on manipulation
c. Practical constraints on manipulation
d. No constraints on manipulation

SET B	**RESPONSE**
1. Does the use of certain tampons cause toxic shock syndrome?	_____
2. Does heroin addiction among mothers affect Apgar scores of infants?	_____
3. Is the age of a hemodialysis patient related to the incidence of the disequilibrium syndrome?	_____
4. What body positions aid respiratory function?	_____
5. Do oral contraceptives cause breast cancer?	_____
6. Does fatigue cause depression in HIV patients?	_____
7. Does the use of touch by nursing staff affect patient morale?	_____
8. Does a nurse's gender affect his or her salary and rate of promotion?	_____
9. Does extreme athletic exertion in young women cause amenorrhea?	_____
10. Does assertiveness training affect a psychiatric nurse's job performance?	_____

B. Completion Exercises

Write the words or phrases that correctly complete the following sentences.

1. The aspect of research design that concerns whether or not there is an intervention involves the distinction between _____ and _____ designs.

2. Researchers generally design their studies to include one or more type of _____ to make their results more interpretable.

3. Designs for qualitative studies tend to be highly _____ .

4. When data are collected at a single point in time, the design is

   _____ .

5. Longitudinal studies conducted to determine the long-term outcome of some condition or intervention are called _____ .

6. In an experiment, the researcher manipulates the _____ variable.

7. The manipulation that the researcher introduces is referred to as the experimental _____ .

8. Randomization is performed so that groups will be formed without

   _____ .

9. Another term for randomization is _____ .

10. When more than one independent variable is being simultaneously manipulated by the researcher, the design is referred to as a(n) _____ .

11. The most typical method of randomization is through the use of a(n)

    _____ .

12. When data are gathered before the institution of some treatment, the initial data gathering is referred to as the _____ .

13. When neither the subjects nor the individuals collecting data know in which group a subject is participating, the procedures are called

    _____ .

14. Each factor in an experimental design must have two or more

    _____ .

15. Another term used for a repeated measures design is a(n) _____ design.

16. A primary objective of a true experiment is to enable the researcher to infer

    _____ .

17. When a true experimental design is not used, the control group is usually referred to as the _____ group.

18. A research design that lacks the controls of a quasi-experiment but involves an intervention is referred to as a(n) _____ design.

19. A quasi-experimental design that involves repeated observations over time is referred to as a(n) _____ design .

20. The difficulty with a nonequivalent control group design is that the experimental and comparison groups cannot be assumed to be _____ before the intervention.

21. When no variable is manipulated in a study, the research is called _____ .

22. Ex post facto research is also referred to as _____ research.

23. Correlation does not prove _____ .

24. A prospective design is more rigorous in elucidating casual relationships than a(n) _____ design.

25. A retrospective design that involves a comparison of a group with a specified disease or condition with another group without the disease or condition is called a(n) _____ design.

26. The _____ rate is the rate at which new cases develop in a specified time interval.

27. The fallacy of "post hoc, ergo propter hoc" lies in an assumption that one thing caused another simply because the presumed cause _____ the presumed effect.

28. _____ is the estimated risk of "caseness" for one group in comparison to that for another.

C. Study Questions

1. Define the following terms. Compare your definition with the definition in Chapter 8 or in the glossary of the textbook.

   a. Research design: _____

   _____

   b. Cross-sectional design: _____

   _____

c. Longitudinal design: _____

_____

d. Panel study: _____

_____

e. Attrition: _____

_____

f. Manipulation: _____

_____

g. Randomization: _____

_____

h. Control group: _____

_____

i. Solomon four-group design: _____

_____

j. Interaction effects: _____

_____

k. Cluster randomization: _____

_____

l. Hawthorne effect: _____

_____

m. Double-blind procedures_____

_____

n. Quasi-experiment: _____

_____

o. Rival hypothesis: _____

_____

p. Correlational research: _____

_____

q. Retrospective design: _____

_____

r. Prospective design: _____

_____

s. Natural experiment: _____

_____

t. Univariate descriptive study: _____

_____

u. Point prevalence rate: _____

_____

v. Relative risk: _____

_____

w. Self-selection: _____

_____

x. Counterfactual: _____

_____

2. Suppose you wanted to study self-esteem among successful dieters who lost 20 or more pounds and maintained their weight loss for at least 6 months. Specify at least two different types of comparison strategies that might provide a useful comparative context for this study.

3. Suppose you wanted to study the coping strategies of AIDS patients at different points in the progress of the disease. Design a cross-sectional study to research this question, describing how subjects would be selected. Now design a longitudinal study to research the same problem. Identify the strengths and weaknesses of the two approaches.

4. Below are 20 subjects who have volunteered for a study of the effects of noise on pulse rate. Ten must be assigned to the low-volume group and 10 to a high-volume group. Use the random numbers in Table 8-2 of the text to assign subjects randomly to groups and groups to treatments.

L. Bentley	M. McGowan
L. Boehm	A. Messenger
D. Chorna	U. Moore
H. Dann	P. Morrill
E. Gordon	C. O'Dea
R. Greenberg	A. Petty
C. Hetsko	J. Riffin
J. Harte	V. Rotan
S. Kulli	H. Seidler
P. Labovitz	R. Smalling

Assume all participants in the first column above are in their 20s and all those in the second column are in their 30s. How good a job did your randomization do in terms of equalizing the experimental and control groups according to age? Add 10 more names to each age group and assign these additional 20 subjects to the two treatment groups. Now compare the low-volume and high-volume groups in terms of the age distribution. Did doubling the sample size improve the distribution of subjects' ages within the two volume-level groups?

5. A nurse researcher found a relationship between teenagers' level of knowledge about birth control and their level of sexual activity. That is, teenagers with higher levels of sexual activity knew more about birth control than teenagers with less sexual activity. Suggest at least three interpretations for this finding. Is this a research problem that is *inherently* nonexperimental? Why or why not?

6. Indicate which of the following variables *inherently* can or cannot be manipulated by a researcher.*

   a. Age at onset of obesity _____

   b. Amount of auditory stimulation _____

   c. Number of cigarettes smoked _____

   d. Infant's birth weight _____

   e. Blood type _____

   f. Preoperative anxiety _____

   g. Type of nursing curriculum _____

   h. Attitudes toward evidence-based nursing practice _____

   i. Nurses' shift assignments _____

   j. Type of birth control method used _____

   k. Mother–infant bonding _____

   l. Use of atrioventricular shunt versus atrioventricular fistula _____

   m. Fluid intake _____

   n. Morale of dying patients' family members _____

7. Refer to the 10 hypotheses in Exercises C.5 and C.6 of Chapter 4 (page 42). Indicate below whether these hypotheses could be tested using an experimental/quasi-experimental approach, a nonexperimental approach, or both.

*Remember that *manipulation* does not refer to whether or not the variable can be *affected* by a researcher; it refers to the researcher's ability to randomly assign individuals to different levels of the variable or to different groups.

Experimental/ Quasi-Experimental	Nonexperimental	Both
5a. _____	_____	_____
5b. _____	_____	_____
5c. _____	_____	_____
5d. _____	_____	_____
5e. _____	_____	_____
6a. _____	_____	_____
6b. _____	_____	_____
6c. _____	_____	_____
6d. _____	_____	_____
6e. _____	_____	_____

8. The following study was a double-blind experiment. Review the design for this study, and comment on the appropriateness of the double-blind procedures. What biases was the researcher trying to avoid? Was she successful?

   Macke, J. (2001). Analgesia for circumcision: Effects on newborn behavior and mother/infant interaction. *Journal of Obstetric, Gynecologic, and Neonatal Nursing, 30,* 507–514.

9. Suppose that you were interested in testing the hypothesis that regular ingestion of aspirin reduced the risk of colon cancer. Describe how such a hypothesis could be tested using a retrospective design. Now describe a prospective design for the same study. Compare the strengths and weaknesses of the two approaches.

D. Application Exercises

1. Here is a brief description of the design of a fictitious study. Read the description of the research design and then respond to the questions that follow.

   Marro (2003) hypothesized that aging negatively affects intellectual capacity and motor responsivity. To test this hypothesis, she randomly selected the names of 250 men aged 70 years or older; 250 men in their 50s; and 250 men in their 30s from the residents living in a mid-sized city in Illinois. Marro realized that intellectual capacity is sometimes correlated with social class. Furthermore, mortality rates vary by social class. Therefore, the subjects were selected in such a way that half in each group were from lower-income households (annual household incomes of $30,000 or less) and half were from higher-income households (annual household incomes over $30,000). The basic design for the analysis, therefore, was as follows:

| | AGE GROUP | | |
INCOME GROUP	30s	50s	70s
≤ $30,000			
> $30,000			

The 750 individuals were administered an individual intelligence test that measured verbal aptitude, problem solving, quantitative skills, spatial aptitude, and overall intelligence. Participants also were given various reaction-time tests. The analysis of the data revealed that, as hypothesized, scores on the intelligence measures declined with age in both income groups. Except on the measure of verbal aptitude, the subjects in their 30s scored highest, and those in their 70s scored lowest on the subtests of intellectual capacity and on overall intelligence. The same pattern was observed for reaction time. Marro concluded that the aging process causes deterioration of both intellectual and motor capacity.

Review and critique Marro's study. Suggest alternative designs or other modifications for testing the researcher's hypothesis. To assist you in your critique, here are some guiding questions:

    a. Is this design experimental or nonexperimental; cross-sectional or longitudinal; structured or flexible; between subjects or within subjects?

    b. What comparisons, if any, were planned in this study?

    c. What problems, if any, does this design pose in terms of testing the hypothesis? What design might be more appropriate? What difficulties would the researcher have had in implementing your recommended design?

    d. What extraneous variables did the researcher identify, and how were they controlled? What extraneous variables do you think should have been controlled but were not? Why might the researcher have decided not to control these variables?

2. Below are several suggested research articles. Read the introductory and methods sections of one or more of these articles, and respond to the questions in Exercise D.1 in terms of these actual research studies.

- Drake, D. A. (2001). A longitudinal study of physical activity and breast cancer prediction. *Cancer Nursing, 24,* 371–371.
- Johnson, C. C., Li, D., Perry, C. L., Elder, J. P., Feldman, H. A., Kelder, S. H., & Stone, E. J. (2002). Fifth through eighth grade longitudinal predictors of tobacco use among a racially diverse cohort. *Journal of School Health, 72,* 58–64.
- Maloni, J. A., Kane, J. H., Suen, L. J., & Wang, K. K. (2002). Dysphoria among high-risk pregnant hospitalized women on bed rest: A longitudinal study. *Nursing Research, 51,* 92–99.

- McCrone, S., Lenz, E., Tarzian, A., & Perkins S. (2001). Anxiety and depression: incidence and patterns in patients after coronary artery bypass graft surgery. *Applied Nursing Research, 14,* 155–164.
- Morse, G. G., & House, J. W. (2001). Changes in Meniere's disease responses as a function of the menstrual cycle. *Nursing Research, 50,* 286–292.

3. Below is a brief description of the research design for a fictitious study. Read the summary and then respond to the questions that follow.

   Piekarz (2002) wanted to test the effectiveness of a new relaxation/biofeedback intervention on menopause symptoms. She invited clients of an outpatient clinic who complained of severe hot flashes to participate in the study. The 30 women who agreed to participate were asked to record, every day for 1 week before their treatment, the frequency and duration of their hot flashes. During the intervention, which involved six 1-hour sessions over a 3-week period, the women again recorded their symptoms. Then, 4 weeks after the treatment, the women were asked to record their hot flashes over a 5-day period. At the end of the study, Piekarz found that both the frequency and average duration of the hot flashes had been significantly reduced in this sample of women. She concluded that her new treatment was an effective alternative to estrogen replacement therapy in treating menopausal hot flashes.

   Review and critique this study. Suggest alternative designs for testing the effectiveness of the treatment. To assist you in your critique, here are some guiding questions:

   a. What are the independent and dependent variables in this study?
   b. Is the design described above experimental, quasi-experimental, or preexperimental?
   c. The investigator concluded that the outcome (i.e., the reduction in the frequency and duration of the women's hot flashes) was attributable to the experimental treatment. Can you offer one or more alternative explanations to account for the outcome? Discuss the inference of causality in the context of this research design.
   d. If you have identified any weaknesses in the design of this research, suggest a modified design that would improve the study. In what way does your new design eliminate the problems of the original design?

4. Below are several suggested research articles. Read one or more of these articles, and respond to questions a through d from Question D.3 in terms of these actual research studies.

   - Adachi, K., Shimada, M., & Usui, A. (2003). The relationship between the parturient's positions and perceptions of labor pain intensity. *Nursing Research, 52,* 47–56.
   - George, E. L., Hofa L. A., Boujoukos, A., & Zullo, T. G. (2002). Effect of positioning on oxygenation in single-lung transplant recipients. *American Journal of Critical Care, 11,* 66–75.

- Hill, A. S., Kurkowski, T. B., & Garcia, J. (2000). Oral support measures used in feeding the preterm infant. *Nursing Research, 49,* 2–10.
- Modrcin-Talbott, M. A., Harrison, L. L., Groer, M. W., & Younger, M. S. (2003). the biobehavioral effects of gentle human touch on preterm infants. *Nursing Science Quarterly, 16,* 60–67.
- Varda, K. E., & Behnke, R. S. (2000). The effect of timing of initial bath on newborn's temperature. *Journal of Obstetric, Gynecologic, and Neonatal Nursing, 29,* 27–32.

5. Another brief summary of the research design for a fictitious study is presented next. Read the summary and then answer the questions that follow.

Sephas (2003) hypothesized that the paucity of socioemotional supports among the elderly results in a high level of chronic health problems and low morale. She tested this hypothesis by interviewing a sample of 250 residents of one community who were aged 65 years and older. The respondents were randomly selected from a list of town residents. Sephas used several measures regarding the availability of socioemotional supports: (1) whether the respondent lived with any kin; (2) whether the respondent had any living children who resided within 30 minutes away; (3) the total number of interactions the respondent had had in the previous week with kin not residing in his or her household; and (4) the number of close friends in whom the respondent felt he or she could confide. Based on responses to the various questions on social support, respondents were classified in one of three groups: low social support, moderate social support, and high social support.

In a 6-month follow-up interview, Sephas collected information from 214 respondents about the frequency and intensity of the respondents' illnesses in the preceding 6 months, their hospitalization record, overall satisfaction with life, and attitudes toward their own aging. The data analysis revealed that the low-support group had significantly more health problems, lower life satisfaction ratings, and lower acceptance of their aging than the other two groups. Sephas concluded that the availability of social supports resulted in better physical and mental adjustment to old age.

Review and critique this study. Suggest alternative designs for testing the researcher's hypothesis. To assist you in your critique, here are some guiding questions:

    a. What are the independent and dependent variables in this study?
    b. Is this research nonexperimental? If so, is it *inherently* nonexperimental? Why or why not? If so, what *type* of nonexperimental research is it?
    c. Examine the criteria for causality presented in Chapter 8 of the text. Does this study meet all the criteria for establishing causality?
    d. The researcher concluded that her independent variable "caused" certain outcomes. Can you offer two or more alternative explanations to account for the outcome?
    e. Consider your responses to parts b and c above. If you have identified any weaknesses in the design of this research, suggest modifications that would improve the study design.

6. Below are several suggested research articles. Read the introductory and method sections of one or more of these articles, and respond to questions a through e from Question D.3 in terms of these actual research studies.

- Kozuki, Y., & Frowlicher, E. S. (2003). Lack of awareness and nonadherence in schizophrenia. *Western Journal of Nursing Research, 25,* 57–74.
- Lampic, C., Thurfjell, E., Bergh, J., Carolsson, M., & Sjödén, P. (2002). Life values before versus after a breast cancer diagnosis. *Research in Nursing & Health, 25,* 89–98.
- Mastaglia, B., & Kristjanson, L. J. (2001). Factors influencing women's decisions for choice of surgery for Stage I and Stage II breast cancer in Western Australia. *Journal of Advanced Nursing, 35,* 836–847.
- Millner, V. S., & Eichold, B. H. (2001). Body piercing and tattooing perspectives. *Clinical Nursing Research, 10,* 424–441.
- Scherbring, M. (2002). Effect of caregiver perception of preparedness on burden in an oncology population. *Oncology Nursing Forum, 29,* E70–76.

E. Special Projects

1. Suppose you wanted to compare premature and full-term babies in terms of their physical and cognitive development at 5 years of age. Describe a broad design for such a study, being careful to indicate the number of times data would be collected. Discuss the rationale for your design.

2. A nurse researcher is interested in testing the effect of packing sugar on a wound on the wound-healing process. Describe a design you would recommend for this problem, being careful to indicate what extraneous variables you would need to control and how you would control them, and what comparisons could be made to enhance the interpretability of the results. Discuss the rationale for your decisions.

3. Suppose you wanted to test the hypothesis that a regular regimen of exercise reduces blood pressure, improves cardiovascular efficiency, and increases coronary circulation. Design a quasi-experiment to test the hypothesis. Evaluate this design in terms of the ability to make causal inferences. Design a true experiment to test the same hypothesis, and compare the kinds of conclusions that can be drawn with this design with those from the quasi-experiment. Describe how you might design a correlational study to test the same hypothesis.

4. Suppose that you wanted to test the hypothesis that gingko improves memory in postmenopausal women. Describe how such a hypothesis could be tested using a retrospective design. Now describe a prospective design for the same study. Compare the strengths and weaknesses of the two approaches. Could an experimental or quasi-experimental design be used? Why or why not?

CHAPTER **9**

Enhancing Rigor in Quantitative Research

A. Matching Exercises

Match each validity threat from Set B with a phrase from Set A that indicates the nature of the threat. Indicate the letter corresponding to your response next to each statement in Set B.

SET A
a. Internal validity
b. External validity
c. Neither internal nor external validity

SET B	**RESPONSE**
1. Selection	_____
2. Maturation	_____
3. Manipulation	_____
4. Novelty effect	_____
5. Replication	_____
6. Testing	_____
7. Hawthorne effect	_____
8. Experimenter effect	_____
9. Blocking	_____
10. Mortality	_____

B. Completion Exercises

Write the words or phrases that correctly complete the following sentences.

1. The environment should be controlled by the researcher insofar as possible by maximizing _____ in the research conditions.

2. In crossover designs, the technique of _____ can be used to rule out ordering effects.

3. Using the principle of homogeneity to control extraneous variables limits the _____ of the findings.

4. When an extraneous variable is dealt with in a randomized block design, it is essentially treated as another _____ variable.

5. When the technique of _____ is used, a subject in one group is paired with a subject in another group with respect to the extraneous variable being controlled.

6. When comparison groups are made comparable overall with regard to extraneous variables (rather than on a subject-by-subject basis), the design may be referred to as _____.

7. One technique of statistical control is _____.

8. A variable that is especially powerful to control is a _____ measure of the dependent variable.

9. _____ validity is the ability of the design to detect true relationships among variables.

10. A design that maximizes the variability in the dependent variable that can be attributed to the independent variable is enhancing the _____ of the study.

11. When comparison groups are designed to be as different as possible, the _____ of the design is enhanced.

12. A procedure that involves including members of a treatment group only if they did, in fact, receive the intervention is called _____.

13. _____ validity is the extent to which researchers can conclude that the independent variable (and not something else) caused variation in the dependent variable.

14. The differential loss of subjects from comparison groups results in the threat known as _____ .

15. Changes that occur as the result of time passing rather than as a result of an intervention represent the threat of _____ .

16. Events concurrent with the institution of a treatment that can affect the dependent variable constitute the threat of _____ .

17. The group to whom a researcher *ideally* can generalize the research findings is the _____ population.

18. An inadequate sampling plan can affect the _____ validity of a study.

C. Study Questions

1. Define the following terms. Compare your definition with the definition in Chapter 9 or in the glossary of the textbook.

   a. Constancy of conditions: _____

   _____

   b. Contamination of treatments: _____

   _____

   c. Pair matching: _____

   _____

   d. Balanced design: _____

   _____

   e. Statistical control: _____

   _____

   f. Statistical power: _____

   _____

g. Intention to treat: _____

_____

h. Threats to internal validity: _____

_____

i. Selection threat: _____

_____

j. Mortality threat: _____

_____

k. History threat: _____

_____

l. External validity: _____

_____

m. Accessible population: _____

_____

n. Experimenter effect: _____

_____

o. Placebo effect: _____

_____

p. Contact information: _____

_____

2. Examine the 10 research questions in the first matching exercise of Chapter 8. For each, specify one or more extraneous variables that the researcher might want to control.

1. _____

2. _____

3. _____

4. _____

5. _____

6. _____

7. _____

8. _____

9. _____

10. _____

3. A nurse researcher is interested in comparing the oral versus rectal temperature measurements of febrile adults from three different clinical units twice a day. Could such a study be conducted as a factorial experiment? Why or why not? If yes, what are the factors in the design? Could this study be conducted as a repeated measures design? Why or why not? If yes, how would you counterbalance? Could a randomized block design be used? Why or why not? If yes, what would the blocking variable be?

4. Below is a list of five target populations. For five of them, think of an accessible population (i.e., a population accessible to *you*) that you might be able to use if you were conducting the study. Be as specific (and realistic) as possible.

    a. All pregnant women residing in an urban area

    _____

    b. All high school students applying to schools of nursing

    _____

    c. All cigarette smokers

    _____

    d. All men older than 45 years of age who have had a cardiovascular accident

    _____

    e. All licensed midwives

    _____

5. Suppose you wanted to study the effectiveness of an innovative approach to teaching student nurses how to give subcutaneous injections. In conducting a true experiment for this study, what environmental factors would you want to control with respect to maintaining constancy of conditions?

6. Suppose you were studying the effects of range-of-motion exercises on radical mastectomy patients. You start your experiment with 50 experimental subjects and 50 control subjects. Your intervention requires experimental subjects to come for daily sessions over a 2-week period, while control subjects come only once at the end of 2 weeks. Your final group sizes are 40 for the experimental group and 49 for the control group. The results of your study indicate that the experimental group did better in raising the arm of the affected side above head level. What effects, if any, do you think the subject attrition might have on the internal validity of your study?

D. Application Exercises

1. Below is a brief description of the research design for a fictitious study. Read the summary and then respond to the questions that follow.

> Fruci (2003) investigated the relationship between the use of intrauterine contraceptive devices (IUDs) and the incidence of pelvic inflammatory disease (PID) in a sample of urban women. The data were gathered from the gynecology departments of four health centers (one university, one city hospital, one health maintenance organization, and one consortium of private gynecologists). Fruci obtained the records of 600 women—150 from each facility—who were diagnosed within the previous 12 months as having PID. She also obtained the records of 150 women who had come to each of the facilities for some other purpose and who had no record of having had PID within the 12-month period before their focal visit. The two groups of 600 women (the PID and non-PID group) were matched in terms of age (within a 5-year age range of under 20, 20–25, 26–29, 30–35, and so forth) and marital status (currently married or not married). For each of the 1200 women, the records were examined to determine whether they had had an IUD inserted within 2 years before their focal visit. For those women for whom no determination could be made based on the records of the facility, brief telephone interviews were administered to obtain the needed information (30 women who could not be reached were replaced with other women to maintain the sample size). The data revealed that 122 women in the PID group (20.3%), compared with 74 women in the non-PID group (12.3%), had used an IUD, a significant group difference. Based on this analysis, Fruci concluded that use of an IUD was a cause of PID in this sample.

Review and critique this study. Suggest alternative designs for examining the research problem. To assist you in your critique, here are some guiding questions:

   a. Is this research nonexperimental? If so, is it *inherently* nonexperimental? Why or why not?
   b. Evaluate the internal validity of the study. What threats to its internal validity, if any, are posed?
   c. Examine the criteria for causality presented in Chapter 8 of the text. Does this study meet all the criteria for establishing causality?
   d. The researcher concluded that her independent variable (use of the IUD) "caused" a certain outcome (incidence of PID). Can you offer two or more alternative explanations to account for the outcome?
   e. What extraneous variables did the researcher identify, and by what method were they controlled? How else might those variables have been controlled?
   f. What extraneous variables do you think *should* have been controlled but were not? Why might the researcher have decided *not* to control these variables?
   g. To what extent did the researcher control for the constancy of conditions in this study? Suggest ways in which this aspect of the study could have been improved.

   h. What is the target population of this study? What is the accessible population? How reasonable is it to generalize the results of this study to the target population?

   i. Evaluate the external validity of the study in terms of the "threats" described in Chapter 9. What changes, if any, would you recommend to improve the external validity of the design?

2. Below are several suggested research articles. Read one or more of these articles and respond to questions a through i of Question D.1 in terms of these actual research studies.

   - Kelechi, T. J., Haight , B. K., Herman, J., Michel, Y., Brothers, T., & Edlund, B. (2003). Skin temperature and chronic venous insufficiency. *Journal of Wound Ostomy and Continence Nursing, 30,* 17–24.
   - Moon, J. S., & Cho, K. S. (2001). The effects of handholding on anxiety in cataract surgery patients under local anaesthesia. *Journal of Advanced Nursing, 35,* 407–415.
   - Smith, M., Casey, L., Johnson, D., Gwede, C., & Riggin, O. Z. (2001). Music as a therapeutic intervention for anxiety in patients receiving radiation therapy. *Oncology Nursing Forum, 28,* 855–862.
   - Whitney, J. D., Salvadalena, G., Higa, L., & Mich, M. (2001). Treatment of pressure ulcers with noncontact normothermic wound therapy: Healing and warming effects. *Journal of WOCN, 28,* 244–252.

3. Below is a brief description of another research design for a fictitious study. Read the summary and then respond to the questions in D.1.

   Kimelberg (2003) studied the efficacy of scheduled nap therapy on the episodes of sleep attacks and symptom severity among 25 narcoleptic patients from a sleep disorder clinic in New York City. The therapy consisted of three scheduled 10-minute naps daily at 10 AM, 1 PM, and 3 PM. Subjects maintained daily sleep diaries in which they recorded time and duration of sleep episodes for 2 weeks prior to treatment, during the 2-week treatment period, and for 2 weeks following treatment. The severity of common narcoleptic symptoms (e.g., sleepiness, sleep paralysis) was also assessed prior to and following treatment. Treatment occurred in a sleep laboratory, with all subjects reporting at 9 AM and being given guidance on scheduled napping. Kimelberg found that the frequency of sleep attacks or the severity of narcoleptic symptoms did not improve over the course of the study and concluded that the intervention was not effective.

4. Below are several suggested research articles. Read one or more of these articles and respond to questions a through i of Question D.1 in terms of these actual research studies.

   - Given, B., Given, C.W., McCorkle, R., Kozachik, S., Cimprich, B., Rahbar, M. H., & Wojcik, C. (2002). Pain and fatigue management: results of a nursing randomized clinical trial. *Oncology Nursing Forum, 29,* 949–956.

- Hamel, C. F., Guse, L. W., Hawranik, P. G., & Bond, J. B. (2002). Advance directives and community-dwelling older adults. *Western Journal of Nursing Research, 24,* 143–158.
- Hattan, J., King, L., & Griffiths, P. (2002). The impact of foot massage and guided relaxation following cardiac surgery: a randomized controlled trial. *Journal of Advanced Nursing, 37,* 199–207.
- McDougall, G.J. (2002). Memory improvement in octogenarians. *Applied Nursing Research, 15,* 2–10.
- Shertzer, K. E., & Keck, J. F. (2002). Music and the PACU environment. *Journal of Perianesthesia Nursing, 16,* 90–102.

E. Special Projects

1. Suppose you wanted to compare the growth patterns of infants whose mothers were heroin addicts with those of infants of nonaddicted mothers. Describe how you would design such a study, being careful to indicate what extraneous variables you would need to control and how you would control them. Identify the major threats to the internal validity of your design.

2. A nurse researcher is interested in testing the effect of a special high-fiber diet on cardiovascular risk factors (e.g., cholesterol level) in adults with a family history of cardiovascular disease. Describe a design you would recommend for this problem, being careful to indicate what extraneous variables you would need to control and how you would control them. Suggest methods of strengthening the power of the design. Identify possible threats to the internal validity of your design.

CHAPTER **10**

Quantitative Research for Various Purposes

A. Matching Exercises

1. Match each feature from Set B with one (or more) of the phrases from Set A that indicates a type of quantitative research. Indicate the letter(s) corresponding to your response next to each statement in Set B.

SET A
a. Clinical trial
b. Evaluation research
c. Methodologic research
d. Survey research
e. Outcomes research
f. Needs assessment

SET B   **RESPONSE**

1. Can involve an experimental design   _____

2. Cost—benefit analyses are one type   _____

3. May involve a study of the link between structures
   and processes   _____

4. Data are always from self-reports   _____

5. The aim is to develop better instruments and procedures
   for research   _____

6. Often designed in a series of phases (I through IV)   _____

7. One approach to doing such studies is called "goal free"   _____

8. Benefits from controls over extraneous variables   _____

9. Can be designed so that data are analyzed sequentially   _____

10. An indicators approach may be used in this type of research _____

B. Completion Exercises

Write the words or phrases that correctly complete the following sentences.

1. Phase III trials may be referred to as _____.

2. In sequential clinical trials, pairs are compared using measures of _____.

3. In classical evaluation research, behavioral objectives focus on the behavior of the _____ of a program, not the agents.

4. A _____ analysis provides descriptive information about how a policy or program works in practice.

5. Impact analyses use an experimental or quasi-experimental design to determine a program's _____.

6. Two types of cost analyses are _____ and _____.

7. Intervention research involves the development of a(n) _____ during the planning phase of the project.

8. _____ is undertaken to document the effectiveness of health care services.

9. In Donabedian's original model of health care appraisal, the three factors that were emphasized were _____, _____, and _____.

10. Replication studies that are exact duplicates of earlier studies are called _____ replication, but when precise duplication is not sought, they may be called _____ replication.

11. Methodologic research is so named because it is research conducted for the purpose of developing or refining research _____ .

12. In surveys, _____ interviews are less expensive than in-person interviews.

13. A survey conducted with an entire population is a(n) _____.

14. A researcher who initially attempts to collect survey data via the telephone, but then uses a personal interview if the telephone does not result in an interview is using a(n) _____ strategy.

15. The method of collecting needs assessment data by questioning knowledgeable individuals is known as the _____ approach.

16. When a researcher analyzes data as a secondary analysis and either aggregates or disaggregates the data differently than in the original research, we say that there has been a change in the _____ .

17. The procedure known as _____ uses statistical procedures to aggregate findings from prior studies, using each study as the unit of analysis.

18. Respondents in a Delphi survey are referred to as a(n) _____ .

C. Study Questions

1. Define the following terms. Compare your definition with the definition in Chapter 10 or in the glossary of the textbook.

   a. Clinical trial:_____

   _____

   b. Sequential clinical trial: _____

   _____

   c. Stopping rules: _____

   _____

   d. Policy research:_____

   _____

   e. Summative evaluation:_____

   _____

   f. Impact analysis:_____

   _____

   g. Subgroup analysis: _____

   _____

   h. Cost—benefit analysis: _____

   _____

   i. Intervention research: _____

   _____

   j. Nursing minimal data set: _____

   _____

   k. Systematic extension replication: _____

   _____

   l. Survey research: _____

   _____

   m. Needs assessment: _____

   _____

   n. Secondary analysis: _____

   _____

   o. Meta-analysis: _____

   _____

   p. Methodologic research: _____

   _____

2. In what ways are impact analyses and Phase III clinical trials similar and different?

   _____

   _____

   _____

3. Listed below are several programs or policies that could be evaluated. For each, think of one or more objectives that such a program might have that would be amenable to evaluation, and state them as *behavioral* objectives. Remember that it is the intended behavior of program *beneficiaries* that must be specified.

   a. A continuing education workshop on new techniques in monitoring intracranial pressure

   _____

   _____

b. A seminar to improve nurses' instructions to dialysis patients regarding the hygienic care of their shunts

_____

_____

c. A crisis intervention program for rape victims

_____

_____

d. A program to educate primiparas with regard to breastfeeding their infants

_____

_____

4. Consider a client group of interest to you. Suggest an approach for conducting a needs assessment for this group. What needs would you focus on for this group?

5. Read the following research report. Indicate what you might do to undertake a virtual replication of this study. What aspects of the study would you change, and why?

   Pack-Mabien, A., Labbe, E., Herbert, D., & Haynes, J. (2001). Nurses' attitudes and practices in sickle cell pain management. *Applied Nursing Research, 14,* 187—192.

6. Suppose you were interested in studying the research questions below by conducting a survey. For each, indicate whether you would recommend using a personal interview, a telephone interview, or a questionnaire to collect the data. What is your rationale?

   a. What are the coping strategies and behaviors of newly widowed individuals?

   _____

   b. Are the rural elderly more socially isolated that the urban elderly?

   _____

   c. What type of nursing communications do presurgical patients find most helpful?

   _____

   d. What is the relationship between a teenager's health-risk appraisal and their risk-taking behavior (e.g., smoking, unprotected sex, drug use)?

   _____

e. What are the health-promoting activities pursued by inner-city single mothers?

_____

f. How is employment of parents affected by the health or disability of a child?

_____

7. Are the problems that survey researchers address usually amenable to experimentation? Why or why not?

D. Application Exercises

1. A brief summary of a fictitious survey study is presented next. Read the summary and then answer the questions that follow.

> Walp (2002) studied the contraceptive practices of university students at three large Midwestern universities. In addition to obtaining descriptive information, he wanted to test the hypothesis that students who report favorable experiences with health care personnel relating to contraceptives are more likely than those with unfavorable experiences to practice birth control effectively. A random sample of 500 students from each university was sent a mailed questionnaire. A total of 715 usable questionnaires were returned.
>
> The survey questionnaire included questions on sexual experience, contraceptive use history, perceived ease of access to birth control, feelings about seeking out contraceptive information, knowledge of on-campus contraceptive services, and experiences with health care personnel related to contraception. The questionnaire also asked about the students' age, ethnicity, year in college, major, father's occupation, marital status, religion, and grade point average.
>
> Walp's data revealed that while most students were sexually experienced, only about half had used any birth control during their last intercourse. About 60% of the sexually active students had had a contact with health care personnel relating to contraceptives, and of these, 70% described their experience in positive terms. In comparing those who had had favorable and unfavorable experiences, Walp found that a significantly higher percentage of those with a favorable than unfavorable experience (68% versus 42%, respectively) had used some form of contraceptive at last intercourse. He concluded that a favorable experience with health care personnel leads to better contraceptive utilization. He speculated that those with more positive experiences were better informed about and more accepting of contraception than those with negative experiences and hence practiced birth control more conscientiously.

Review and critique this study. Suggest alternative methods for conducting this research. To assist you in your critique, here are some guiding questions:

a. Is this research nonexperimental? If so, is it *inherently* nonexperimental? Why or why not?

    b. What type of research study is this, in terms of the types discussed in this chapter? Could the same research problem be studied using an alternative approach (i.e., one of the other types of research discussed in the chapter)?

    c. Examine the criteria for causality presented in Chapter 8 of the text. Does this study meet all the criteria for establishing causality?

    d. The researcher concluded that the independent variable "caused" a certain outcome. Can you offer alternative explanations to account for the outcome?

    e. Prepare two or three hypotheses that you could test in a secondary analysis of this researcher's data.

2. Below are several suggested research articles. Skim one or more of these articles and respond to questions a through e from Question D.1 in terms of this actual research study.

- Erlen, J. A., Sereika, S. M., Cook, R. L., & Hunt, S. C. (2002). Adherence to antiretroviral therapy among women with HIV infection. *Journal of Obstetric, Gynecologic, and Neonatal Nursing, 31,* 470–477.
- King, K. B., Quinn, J. R., Delehanty, J. M., Rizzo, S., Eldredge, D. H., Caufield, L., & Ling, F. S. (2002). Perception of risk for coronary heart disease in women undergoing coronary angiography. *Heart & Lung, 31,* 246–252.
- Price, J. H., Telljohann, S. K., Dake, J. A., Marsico, L., & Zyla, C. (2002). Urban elementary school students' perceptions of fighting behavior and concerns for personal safety. *Journal of School Health, 72,* 184–191.
- Stacey, D., DeGrasse, C., & Johnston, L. (2002). Addressing the support needs of women at high risk for breast cancer: Evidence-based care by advanced practice nurses. *Oncology Nursing Forum, 29,* E77–84.
- Wood, F. G. (2002). Ethnic differences in exercise among adults with diabetes. *Western Journal of Nursing Research, 24,* 502–515.

E. Special Projects

1. Find an example of an outcomes research study. On what aspect of the structure-process-client-outcomes nexus did the researchers focus? Suggest ways to extend the research by incorporating at least one other factor.

2. Generate five hypotheses that could be tested using survey data from the study described in Question D.1.

CHAPTER **11**

Qualitative Research Design and Approaches

A. Matching Exercises

1. Match each descriptive statement from Set B with one of the research traditions from Set A. Indicate the letter corresponding to your response next to each item in Set B.

SET A

a. Ethnography
b. Phenomenology
c. Grounded theory
d. Ethnography, phenomenology, and
   grounded theory

SET B   **RESPONSE**

1. Is rooted in a philosophical tradition developed by Husserl
   and Heidegger   _____

2. Studies both broadly defined cultures and more narrowly
   defined ones   _____

3. Uses qualitative data to address questions of interest   _____

4. Is an approach to the study of social processes and social
   structures   _____

5. Is concerned with the lived experiences of humans   _____

6. Strives to achieve an emic perspective on the members of a
   group   _____

7. Is associated with a research tradition called hermeneutics   _____

8. Uses a procedure referred to as constant comparison   _____

9. Stems from a discipline other than nursing   _____

10. Developed by the sociologists Glaser and Strauss   _____

B. Completion Exercises

Write the words or phrases that correctly complete the following sentences.

1. The design for a qualitative study is often called a(n) _____ design.

2. Qualitative researchers are often adept at performing many diverse tasks and are sometimes referred to as _____.

3. The disciplinary roots of ethnography is _____ ; of ethology is _____; and of ethnomethodology is _____ .

4. Ethnographic research focuses on human _____.

5. An ethnographic study of a Peruvian village would be called a _____, while an ethnographic study of a ward in a psychiatric hospital would be called a _____.

6. The concept _____ is frequently used by ethnographers to describe the researcher's significant role in interpreting a culture.

7. Phenomenologic research focuses on the _____ of phenomena as experienced by people.

8. Phenomenologists study the various aspects of the lived experience, including lived space or _____; lived body or _____; lived time or _____; or lived human relations or _____.

9. Bracketing can be enhanced by keeping detailed notes in a(n) _____.

10. Interpretive phenomenology is referred to as _____.

11. The primary purpose of _____ is to generate comprehensive explanations of phenomena that are grounded in reality.

12. In a grounded theory study, the technique referred to as _____ is used to compare new data with previously collected data to identify commonalities and refine categories.

13. Substantive grounded theory can serve as a springboard for _____, which is a higher level of theory.

14. _____is the systematic collection, evaluation, and synthesis of data relating to past occurrences.

15. A newspaper article written in 1969 about the role of nurses in the Vietnam War would be considered a _____ source.

16. Archival materials can be accessed through _____.

17. In-depth investigations of a single entity, such as an individual or a group, are referred to as _____.

18. _____ analysis focuses on *stories* about people and how they make sense of their lives.

19. A procedure known as _____ involves steps for translating qualitative findings into nursing interventions.

20. Integration of qualitative findings on a topic is increasingly being accomplished through a procedure known as _____.

21. Research conducted within the framework known as _____ is action oriented, designed to transform social groups and inspire enlightened self-knowledge.

22. In _____, researchers work closely with participants, often oppressed or vulnerable groups, to produce action for improvements.

C. Study Questions

1. Define the following terms. Compare your definition with the definition in the glossary or in Chapter 11 of the textbook.

    a. Bricolage: _____

    _____

b. Discourse analysis: _____

_____

c. Hermeneutics: _____

_____

d. Symbolic interaction: _____

_____

e. Emic perspective: _____

_____

f. Etic perspective: _____

_____

g. Autoethnography: _____

_____

h. Ethnonursing research: _____

_____

i. Being-in-the-world: _____

_____

j. Bracketing: _____

_____

k. Historical research: _____

_____

l. External criticism: _____

_____

m. Internal criticism: _____

_____

n. Descriptive qualitative study: _____

_____

o. Critical ethnography: _____

_____

p. Feminist research: _____

_____

2. For each of the following research questions, indicate what type of research tradition would likely guide the inquiry.

   a. What is the social psychological process through which couples adapt to the death of a child?

   _____

   b. How does the culture of a suicide survivors' self-help group contribute to the grieving process?

   _____

   c. What are the power dynamics that arise in conversations between nurses and bed-ridden nursing home patients?

   _____

   d. What is the lived experience of the spousal caretaker of an Alzheimer patient?

   _____

3. Read the following two studies, which exemplify ethnographic and phenomenological studies. What were the central phenomena under investigation? Compare and contrast the methods used in these two studies (e.g., how were data collected? How many study participants were there? To what extent did the design unfold while the researchers were in the field?).

   Ethnographic Study: Mahoney, J. S. (2001). An ethnographic approach to understanding the illness experiences of patients with congestive heart failure and their family members. *Heart & Lung, 30,* 429–436.

   Phenomenological Study: Orshan, S. A., Furniss, K. K., Forst, C., & Santoro, N. (2001). The lived experience of premature ovarian failure. *Journal of Obstetric, Gynecologic, and Neonatal Nursing, 30,* 202–208.

4. Read the following case study:

   Hildingh, C., Fridlund, B., & Segesten, K. (2000). Self-help groups as a support strategy in nursing: a case study. *Rehabilitation Nursing, 25,* 100–104.

Evaluate the extent to which the case study approach was appropriate. What were the drawbacks and benefits of using this approach?

5. Read the following participatory action research study and comment on the roles of participants and researchers:

   Choudhry, U. K., Jandu, S., Mahal, J., Singh, R., Sohi-Pabla, H., & Mutta, B. (2002). Health promotion and participatory action research with South Asian women. *Journal of Nursing Scholarship, 34,* 75–81.

D. Application Exercises

1. Below is a brief description of a qualitative study. Read the summary and then respond to the questions that follow.

> Dake and Kennedy (2003) investigated women who had given their babies up for adoption. They conducted a grounded theory study to examine the process women go through during the first year after they have relinquished their babies. Dake and Kennedy obtained their sample of 28 women through a local support group for women who had given their babies up for adoption. All 28 participants were white, middle/upper-middle class women, ranging in age from 18 to 44. Some of the women (8) were married, but most (20) were single or divorced. The majority of women (18) had no other children, but 10 were mothers with other children at home. Twelve women had made their decision regarding adoption during the first trimester of their pregnancy. Ten women did not decide until their third trimester, and the remaining six women were still struggling with their decision in the hospital after they had delivered their babies. Each of the 28 participants was interviewed once in depth and asked about their postbirth experiences. Interviews, which were tape recorded, ranged in length from 30 to 60 minutes. When all 28 interviews were completed, the constant comparative method was used to analyze the data. Analysis of the transcribed interviews revealed that the basic problem these women had to cope with over the first year after relinquishing their newborns was mourning the child they would never have. Dake and Kennedy reported that four themes emerged from the data analysis that captured the experience of the participants. These four themes were:
>
> 1. Guilt about giving their babies up for adoption consumed the women.
> 2. Women grieved the loss of their children they would never have to love and watch grow up.
> 3. The women were still immersed in agonizing questioning over whether their decision to relinquish their baby was the right one.
> 4. The women had not yet fully come to terms with their choice.

   Review and critique this study. Suggest alternative data collection and analysis approaches. To assist you in your critique, here are some guiding questions.

   a. How structured or flexible was the research design in this study? Comment on how the degree of structure benefited or detracted from the study.
   b. Was this study squarely within one single qualitative tradition? Identify the tradition(s). Was this tradition appropriate, given the research question?
   c. Was the use of a qualitative approach justified, given the researcher's aims? Would a quantitative approach have been appropriate?

2. Below are several suggested research articles of qualitative studies. Read one or more of these articles and respond to parts a to c of Question D.1 in terms of these actual research studies.

   • Arnaud, D. S. (2002). Help-seeking and social support in Japanese sojourners. *Western Journal of Nursing Research, 24,* 295–306.

- Halstead, M. T., & Hull, M. (2001). Struggling with paradoxes: the process of spiritual development in women with cancer. *Oncology Nursing Forum, 28,* 1534–1544.
- Maugham, K., Heyman, B., & Matthews, M. (2002). In the shadow of risk. How men cope with a partner's gynaecological cancer. *International Journal of Nursing Studies, 39,* 27–34.
- Van, P., & Meleis, A. I. (2003). Coping with grief after involuntary pregnancy loss: perspectives of African American women. *Journal of Obstetric, Gynecologic, and Neonatal Nursing, 32,* 28–39.
- Velji, K., & Fitch, M. (2001). The experience of women receiving brachytherapy for gynecologic cancer. *Oncology Nursing Forum, 28,* 743–751.

3. Below is description of a fictitious qualitative study. Read the summary and then respond to the questions in D. 1.

   Kenneth (2003) explored mothers' experiences of hydrotherapy in labor. Quantitative research had revealed that maternal anxiety and pain were significantly reduced by hydrotherapy. No qualitative research had been undertaken to examine the mothers' experiences with this procedure during their labor, so Kenneth conducted a descriptive phenomenological study of this phenomenon. Because not many local hospitals were offering hydrotherapy, Kenneth had difficulty finding mothers who fit the sample criteria, even though she had advertised the study in the newspaper. Four mothers comprised her purposive sample. All four women were married, Caucasian, and held doctoral degrees. Each participant was interviewed in her home within 6 weeks after delivery. Interviews were tape recorded and lasted on average 15 minutes. Mothers were asked to respond to the following statement: "Please describe your experience of hydrotherapy during labor in as much detail as you can remember. Describe all your thoughts, feelings, and perceptions that you wish to share." Kenneth did not use a predetermined list of structured questions to guide the interviews. During each of the four interviews, an additional family member happened to be present in the home. Prior to and during data collection, Kenneth kept a journal and used it to help her bracket. In analyzing the data, Kenneth identified three themes describing the essence of mothers' experiences with hydrotherapy during their labor. These themes focused on mothers' experiencing an aura of calmness that surrounded them and a heightened feeling of closeness with their infants. No mention of data saturation was included in the research report.

4. Below are several additional suggested research articles of qualitative studies. Read one or more of these articles and respond to parts a to c of Question D.1 in terms of these actual research studies.

   - Boughton, M. A. (2002). Premature menopause: multiple disruptions between the woman's biological body experience and her lived body. *Journal of Advanced Nursing, 37,* 423–430.
   - Emami, A., Benner, P., & Ekman, S. L. (2001). A sociocultural health model for late-in-life immigrants. *Journal of Transcultural Nursing, 12,* 15–24.

- Freda, M. C., Devine, K. S., & Semelsberger, C. (2003). The lived experience of miscarriage after infertility. *MCN: The American Journal of Maternal/Child Nursing, 28*, 16–23.
- Howell, D., Fitch, M., & Caldwell, B. (2002). The impact of interlink community cancer nurses on the experience of living with cancer. *Oncology Nursing Forum, 29*, 715–723.
- Williams-Barnard, C. L., Mendoza, D. C., & Shippee-Rice, R. V. (2001). The lived experience of college student lesbians' encounters with health care providers. *Journal of Holistic Nursing, 19*, 127–142.

E. Special Projects

1. Prepare a research question that could be investigated within each of the following qualitative traditions:

   a. Ethnographic research:_____

   _____

   b. Phenomenological research: _____

   _____

   c. Grounded theory: _____

   _____

   d. Case study: _____

   _____

   e. Critical theory study: _____

   _____

2. Select one of the research questions from Exercise E.1. Lay out a preliminary plan for undertaking a study to address that question, using the guidelines presented in the section titled "Qualitative Design and Planning."

CHAPTER **12**

Integration of Qualitative and Quantitative Designs

A. Matching Exercises

Match each descriptive statement from Set B with one of the statements from Set A. Indicate the letter corresponding to your response next to each item in Set B.

SET A
a. Qualitative data
b. Quantitative data
c. Both qualitative and quantitative data
d. Neither qualitative nor quantitative data

SET B   **RESPONSE**

1. Should be collected to develop evidence for nursing practice   _____

2. Are especially useful for understanding dynamic processes   _____

3. Are often collected in large-scale surveys   _____

4. Are useful in proving the validity of theories   _____

5. Are usually collected by phenomenological researchers   _____

6. Can profit from triangulation   _____

7. Are often used in tests of causal relationships   _____

8. Can contribute to theoretical insights   _____

9. Require validity checks   _____

10. Tend to be collected from small samples   _____

B. Completion Exercises

Write the words or phrases that correctly complete the following sentences.

1. Qualitative and quantitative data may, for some research problems, be _____ in that they "mutually supply each other's lack."

2. The major conceptual frameworks of nursing demand neither _____ nor _____ data.

3. Progress in a developing area of research tends to be _____ and can profit from multiple feedback loops.

4. A major advantage of integrating different approaches is potential enhance-ments to the study's _____ .

5. A frequent application of multimethod studies is in the development of research _____.

6. In a quantitative study, the inclusion of qualitative data might facilitate the _____ of the findings, and vice versa.

7. When qualitative data collection is embedded in a survey effort, it is often more productive to use a _____ approach.

8. In studies of the effects of complex interventions, qualitative data may be use-ful in addressing the _____ question.

9. A major barrier to multimethod research is _____ biases.

10. Although a multimethod data collection and analysis approach is _____ , it can be argued that the collection of multiple types of data in a single study is efficient.

11. In a(n) _____ design, the qualitative and quantitative portions of the study are implemented as discrete aspects.

12. In a(n) _____ design, the qualitative and quantitative aspects of the study are blended together from the outset.

C. Study Questions

1. Define the following terms. Compare your definition with the definition in Chapter 12 or in the glossary of the textbook.

a. Multimethod research: _____

_____

b. Black box: _____

_____

c. Epistemologic bias: _____

_____

d. Complementarity: _____

_____

e. Triangulation: _____

_____

2. Read one of the following studies, in which qualitative data were gathered and analyzed to address a research question. Suggest ways in which the collection of quantitative data might have enriched the study, strengthened its validity, and/or enhanced its interpretability. (Alternatively, defend the collection of qualitative data exclusively.)

   • Fergus, K. D., Gray, R. E., Fitch, M. I., Labrecque, M., & Phillips, C. (2002). Active consideration: Conceptualizing patient-provided support for spouse caregivers in the context of prostate cancer. *Qualitative Health Research, 12,* 492–514.
   • Reed, D. B., & Claunch, D. T. (2002). Behind the scenes: Spousal coping following permanently disabling injury of farmers. *Issues in Mental Health Nursing, 23,* 231–248.
   • Richer, M. C., & Ezer, H. (2002). Living in it, living with it, and moving on: dimensions of meaning during chemotherapy. *Oncology Nursing Forum, 29,* 113–119.
   • Treat-Jacobson, D., Halverson, S. L., Ratchford, A., Regensteiner, J. G., Lindquist, R., & Hirsch, A. T. (2002). A patient-derived perspective of health-related quality of life with peripheral arterial disease. *Journal of Nursing Scholarship, 34,* 55–60.

3. Read one of the following studies, in which quantitative data were gathered and analyzed to address a research question. Suggest ways in which the collection of qualitative data might have enriched the study, strengthened its validity, or enhanced its interpretability:

   • Artinian, N. T., Magnan, M., Sloan, M., & Lange, M. P. (2002). Self-care behaviors among patients with heart failure. *Heart & Lung, 31,* 161–172.
   • Becker, H., Stuifbergen, A. K., & Gordon, D. (2002). The decision to take hormone replacement therapy among women with disabilities. *Western Journal of Nursing Research, 24,* 264–281.

- Pullen, C., & Noble-Walker, S. (2002). Midlife and older rural women's adherence to U.S. dietary guidelines across stages of change in healthy eating. *Public Health Nursing, 19,* 170–178.
- Walker, L. O., & Kim, M. (2002). Psychosocial thriving during late pregnancy: Relationship to ethnicity, gestational weight gain, and birth weight. *Journal of Obstetric, Gynecologic, and Neonatal Nursing, 31,* 263–274.

D. Application Exercises

1. Below is a brief description of a mixed method study, followed by a critique. Do you agree with this critique? Can you add other comments regarding the study design?

Fictitious Study. Tacy (2003) conducted a study designed to examine the emotional well-being of women who had a mastectomy. Tacy wanted to develop an in-depth understanding of the emotional experiences of women as they recovered from their surgery, including the process by which they handled their fears, their concerns about their sexuality, their levels of anxiety and depression, their methods of coping, and their social supports.

Tacy's basic study design was qualitative, loosely within the grounded theory tradition. She gathered information from a sample of 25 women, primarily by means of in-depth interviews with the women on two occasions. The first interviews were scheduled within 1 month after the surgery. Follow-up interviews were conducted about 12 months after the surgery. Several of the women in the sample participated in a support group, and Tacy attended and made observations at several of those meetings. Additionally, Tacy decided to interview the "significant other" (usually the women's husbands) of most of the women, when she learned that the women's emotional well-being was linked to the manner in which the significant other was reacting to the surgery.

In addition to the rich, in-depth information she gathered, Tacy wanted to be able to better interpret the emotional status of the women. Therefore, at both the original and follow-up interview with the women, she administered a psychological scale known as the Center for Epidemiological Studies Depression Scale (CES-D), a quantitative measure that has scores that can range from 0 to 60. This scale has been widely used in community populations and has "cut-off" scores designating when a person is at risk of clinical depression (i.e., a score of 16 and above).

Tacy's qualitative analysis showed that the basic process underlying psychological recovery from the mastectomy was something she labeled "Gaining by Losing," a process that involved heightened self-awareness and self-respect after an initial period of despair and self-pity. The process also involved, for some, a strengthening of personal relationships with significant others, whereas for others, it resulted in the birth of awareness of fundamental deficiencies in their relationships. The quantitative findings confirmed that a very high percentage of women were at risk of being depressed at 1 month after the mastectomy, but at 12 months, levels of depression were actually modestly lower than in the general population of women.

Critique. In her study, Tacy embedded a quantitative measure into the fieldwork in an interesting manner. The bulk of data were qualitative-in-depth interviews and in-depth observations. However, she also opted to include a well-known measure of depression, which provided her with an important context for interpreting her data. A major advantage of using the CES-D is that this scale has known characteristics in the general population and therefore provided a built-in "comparison group."

Tacy used a flexible design that allowed her to use her initial data to guide her inquiry. For example, she decided to conduct in-depth interviews with significant others when she learned their importance to the women's process of emotional recovery. Tacy did do some advance planning, however, that provided loose guidance. For example, although her questioning undoubtedly evolved while in the field, she had the foresight to realize that to capture a process, she would need to collect data longitudinally. She also made the up-front decision to use the CES-D to supplement the in-depth interviews.

In this study, the findings from the qualitative and quantitative portions of the study were complementary. Both portions of the study confirmed that the women initially had emotional "losses," but eventually they recovered and "gained" in terms of their emotional well-being and their self-awareness. This example illustrates how the validity of study findings can be enhanced by the blending of qualitative and quantitative data. If the qualitative data alone had been gathered, Tacy might not have gotten a good handle on the degree to which the women had actually "recovered" (vis à vis women who had never had a mastectomy). Conversely, if she had collected only the CES-D data, she would have had no insights into the process by which the recovery occurred.

2. Below is a summary of a fictitious multimethod study. Read the summary and then respond to the questions that follow.

Kerls (2003) conducted a study to investigate breastfeeding practices among teenage mothers, who have been found in many studies to be less likely than older mothers to breastfeed. Using birth records from two large hospitals, Kerls contacted 250 young women between 15 and 19 years of age who had given birth in the previous year and invited them to participate in a survey. Those who agreed to participate ($N = 185$) were interviewed by telephone (when possible), using a structured interview that asked about breastfeeding practices, attitudes toward motherhood, availability of social supports, and conflicting demands, such as school attendance or employment. Several psychological scales (including measures of depression and self-esteem) were also administered. Teenagers without a telephone were interviewed in person in their own homes. All the teenagers interviewed at home were also interviewed in greater depth, using a topic guide that focused on such areas as feelings about breastfeeding, the decision-making process that led them to decide whether or not to breastfeed, barriers to breastfeeding, and intentions to breastfeed with any subsequent children. Kerls used the quantitative data to determine the characteristics associated with breastfeeding status and duration. The qualitative data were used to interpret and validate the quantitative findings.

Review and critique this study. Suggest alternative data collection and analysis approaches. To assist you in your critique, here are some guiding questions:

a. Which of the aims of integration, if any, were served by this study?
b. What was the researcher's basic strategy for integration? How effective was this strategy in addressing the aims of integration?

   c. What type of mixed method design was used in this study?

   d. Suggest ways of altering the design of the study and the data collection approach to further promote integrative aims.

   e. Would the study have been stronger if it had involved the collection of quantitative data only? Qualitative data only? Why or why not?

3. Below are several suggested research articles of studies that used an integrated approach. Read one or more of these articles and respond to questions a through e from Question D.1 in terms of these actual research studies.

   - Brauer, D. J. (2001). Common patterns of person-environment interaction in persons with rheumatoid arthritis. *Western Journal of Nursing Research, 23,* 414–430.

   - Collins, S., & Long, A., (2003). Too tired to care? The psychological effects of working with trauma. *Journal of Psychiatric Mental Health Nursing, 10,* 17–27.

   - Hahn, S. J., & Craft-Rosenberg, M. (2002). The disclosure decisions of parents who conceive children using donor eggs. *Journal of Obstetric, Gynecologic, and Neonatal Nursing, 31,* 283–293.

   - Rees, C. E., & Bath, P. A. (2001). Information-seeking behaviors of women with breast cancer. *Oncology Nursing Forum, 28,* 899–907.

   - Wong, F., Ho, M., Chiu, I., Lui, W., Chan, C., & Lee, K. (2002). Factors contributing to hospital readmission in a Hong Kong regional hospital. *Nursing Research, 51,* 40–49.

E. Special Projects

1. Prepare five problem statements that would be amenable to multimethod research.

2. For one of the problems suggested in Exercise E.1, write a two- to three-page description of how the data would be collected and how the use of both qualitative and quantitative data and analysis would strengthen the study.

CHAPTER **13**

Sampling Designs

A. Matching Exercises

1. Match each statement relating to sampling for quantitative studies from Set B with one of the phrases from Set A. Indicate the letter corresponding to your response next to each of the statements in Set B.

SET A
a. Probability sampling
b. Nonprobability sampling
c. Both probability and nonprobability sampling
d. Neither probability nor nonprobability sampling

SET B   **RESPONSE**

1. Includes systematic sampling   _____

2. Allows an estimation of the magnitude of sampling error   _____

3. Guarantees a representative sample   _____

4. Includes quota sampling   _____

5. Requires a sample size of at least 100 subjects   _____

6. Elements are selected by nonrandom methods   _____

7. Can be used with entire populations or with selected strata
   from the populations   _____

8. Used to select populations   _____

9. Elements have an equal chance of being selected   _____

10. Is required when the population is homogeneous   _____

2. Match each type of sampling approach from Set B with one of the phrases from Set A. Indicate the letter corresponding to your response next to each of the statements in Set B.

SET A

a. Sampling approach for quantitative studies
b. Sampling approach for qualitative studies
c. Sampling approach for either quantitative or qualitative studies
d. Sampling approach for neither quantitative nor qualitative studies

SET B   **RESPONSE**

1. Typical case sampling   _____

2. Purposive sampling   _____

3. Cluster sampling   _____

4. Intensity sampling   _____

5. Homogeneous sampling   _____

6. Snowball sampling   _____

7. Stratified random sampling   _____

8. Quota sampling   _____

9. Power sampling   _____

10. Theory-based sampling   _____

B. Completion Exercises

Write the words or phrases that correctly complete the following sentences.

1. A(n)_____ is a subset of the units that comprise the population.

2. The main criterion for evaluating a sample in a quantitative study is its _____ of the population being studied.

3. A sample in a quantitative study would be considered _____ if it systematically over-represented or under-represented a segment of the population.

4. If a population is completely _____ with respect to key attributes, then any sample is as good as any other.

5. Another term used for purposive sample is _____ .

6. Quota samples are essentially convenience samples from selected _____ of the population.

7. Another term for a convenience sampling in a quantitative context is _____ sampling; in a qualitative context, the term _____ sampling is sometimes used for convenience sampling.

8. The most basic type of probability sampling is referred to as _____ sampling.

9. The actual list from which a random sample is taken is referred to as the

   _____.

10. When disproportionate sampling is used, an adjustment procedure known as

    _____ is normally used to estimate population values.

11. Another term used to refer to cluster sampling is _____

    sampling.

12. In systematic samples, the distance between selected elements is referred to as

    the _____ .

13. Differences between population values and sample values are referred to as

    _____ .

14. If a quantitative researcher has confidence in his or her sampling design, the

    results of a study can reasonably be generalized to the _____

    population.

15. As the size of a sample _____, the probability of drawing a

    deviant sample diminishes.

16. If a researcher wanted to draw a systematic sample of 100 from a population

    of 3000, the sampling interval would be _____ .

17. In a qualitative study, sampling decisions are often guided by the potential a

    data source has to be _____ -rich.

18. In _____ sampling, the qualitative researcher deliberately

    reduces variation, while in _____ sampling, the researcher pur-

    posefully selects cases with a wide range of variation on dimensions of interest.

19. _____ sampling involves selecting study participants to

    highlight the average situation.

20. Grounded theory researchers rely on _____ sampling to include

    informants who can best contribute to the emerging theory.

21. Toward the end of the study, qualitative researchers often seek to sample

    _____ or _____ cases.

22. Ethnographers have conversations with dozens of people, but often rely on a

    very small sample of _____ to act as guides to the culture.

C. Study Questions

1. Define the following terms. Compare your definition with the definition in Chapter 13 or in the glossary of the textbook.

   a. Sampling: _____

   _____

   b. Probability sampling: _____

   _____

   c. Nonprobability sampling: _____

   _____

   d. Stratum: _____

   _____

   e. Eligibility criteria: _____

   _____

   f. Convenience sample: _____

   _____

   g. Snowball sampling: _____

   _____

   h. Quota sample: _____

   _____

   i. Random sample: _____

   _____

   j. Disproportionate sampling design: _____

   _____

   k. Cluster sampling: _____

   _____

   l. Systematic sampling: _____

   _____

   m. Screening instrument: _____

   _____

n. Theoretical sampling: _____

_____

o. Maximum variation sampling: _____

_____

p. Extreme case sampling: _____

_____

q. Disconfirming cases: _____

_____

r. Data saturation: _____

_____

2. Using the table of random numbers presented in Table 8-1, select a random sample of 30 names, drawn from a sampling frame of your choice (e.g., a page from a telephone directory, roster of nursing students, a staff list).

3. For each of the following target populations, identify an accessible population (accessible to *you*) that might be used in a study.

TARGET POPULATION	ACCESSIBLE POPULATION
a. All teenagers diagnosed as having scoliosis	_____
b. All nursing home residents over the age of 70 years	_____
c. All rape victims in the United States	_____
d. All individuals with blood type O positive	_____

4. Identify the type of quantitative sampling design used in the following examples:

a. One hundred inmates randomly sampled from a random selection of five federal penitentiaries

_____

b. All the nurses participating in a continuing education seminar

_____

c. Every 20th patient admitted to the emergency department between January and June

_____

d. The first 20 male and the first 20 female patients admitted to the hospital with hypothermia

_____

e. A sample of 250 members randomly selected from a roster of American Nurses' Association members

---

5. Nurse A is planning to study the effects of maternal stress, maternal depression, maternal age, and family economic resources on a child's socioemotional development among both intact and mother-headed families. Nurse B is planning to study body position on patients' respiratory functioning. Describe the kinds of samples that the two nurses would need to use. Which nurse would need the larger sample? Defend your answer.

6. Suppose a qualitative researcher wanted to study the life quality of cancer survivors. Suggest what the researcher might do to obtain a maximum variation sample, a typical case sample, a homogeneous sample, and an extreme case sample.

D. Application Exercises

1. Here is a brief summary of the sampling plan of a fictitious quantitative study. Read the summary and then respond to the questions that follow.

Swain (2002) studied the attitudes of recent nursing school graduates toward evidence-based nursing practice. She was interested in exploring whether attitudes varied in relation to the type of employment or further training the nurses had pursued. She obtained lists of graduates from six schools of nursing in Greater Boston (two schools for each of three different types of programs). She then conducted telephone interviews with 100 graduates from each of the three program types (bachelors, diploma, and associates). Her method was to find, using local telephone directories, the telephone numbers for as many of the names on her lists as she could and to make calls until she had completed 100 interviews with graduates from each group. Thus, her final sample consisted of 300 recently graduated RNs.

Review and critique this research effort. Suggest alternative sampling designs. To assist you in your critique, here are some guiding questions:

a. What type of sampling design was used? Was this design appropriate? Would you recommend a different sampling approach? Why or why not? What are the advantages of the approach used? What are the disadvantages?

b. Identify what you believe to be the target and accessible populations in this study. How representative do you feel the accessible population is of the target population? How representative is the sample of this accessible population? What are some of the possible sources of sampling bias?

c. Were the eligibility criteria for the study clearly spelled out? Did the criteria appear sensible?

d. Did the researcher use a proportionate or disproportionate sampling plan? Is this appropriate? Why or why not?

e. Comment on the size of the sample. Does this sample size appear to be adequate?

2. Below are several suggested research articles. Read the introductory and methods sections of one or more of these articles and respond to questions a through e of Question D.1 in terms of these actual research studies.

- Halcón, L. L., Lifson, A. R., Shew, M., Joseph, M., Hannan, P. J., & Hayman, C. R. (2002). Pap test results among low-income youth: Prevalence of dysplasia and practice implications. *Journal of Obstetric, Gynecologic, and Neonatal Nursing, 31,* 294–304.
- Li, S., & Holm, K. (2003). Physical activity alone and in combination with hormone replacement therapy on vasomotor symptoms in postmenopausal women. *Western Journal of Nursing Research, 25,* 274–288.
- Niederhauser, V. P., Baruffi, G., & Heck, R. (2001). Parental decision-making for the varicella vaccine. *Journal of Pediatric Health Care, 15,* 236–243.
- Salazar, M. K., Kemerer, S., Amann, M. C., & Fabrey, L. J. (2002). Defining the roles and functions of occupational and environmental health nurses: Results of a national job analysis. *AAOHN Journal, 50,* 16–25.
- Stevens, M., Esler, R., & Asher, G. (2002). Transdermal fentanyl for the management of acute pancreatic pain. *Applied Nursing Research, 15,* 102–110.

3. A second brief summary of the sampling strategy of a fictitious study follows. Read the summary and then respond to the questions that follow.

Hunter (2003) conducted an in-depth study of the emotional well-being of couples with fertility impairments. She conducted in-depth interviews with 10 couples who were undergoing infertility treatment in a private clinic, and compared them with 10 couples who had undergone such treatment and were expecting a baby. The interviews with the second group occurred in the fifth month of the pregnancies. In each of the two groups, the researcher began by selecting couples known to have had a range of experience with their fertility treatments (in terms of length and type of treatment and nature of the fertility impairment). Then, after the initial interviews were completed, Hunter recruited additional couples to saturate the theoretical lines that were developing within the data.

Review and critique this research effort. Suggest alternative sampling designs. To assist you in your critique, respond to the questions below.

a. What type of sampling strategy was used?
b. Was this sampling strategy appropriate? Would you recommend a different sampling approach? Why or why not?
c. Comment on the size of the sample. Does this sample size appear to be adequate?

4. Below are several suggested research articles. Read the introductory and methods sections of one or more of these articles and respond to parts a through c of Question D.4 in terms of these actual research studies.

- Coyer, S. M. (2003). Women in recovery discuss parenting while addicted to cocaine. *MCN: The American Journal of Maternal/Child Nursing, 28,* 45–49.
- Friesen, P., Pepler, C., & Hunter, P. (2002). Interactive family learning following a cancer diagnosis. *Oncology Nursing Forum, 29,* 981–987.
- Jones, P. S., Zhang, X. E., Jaceldo-Siegl, K., & Meleis, A. I. (2002). Caregiving between two cultures: An integrative experience. *Journal of Transcultural Nursing, 13,* 202–209.
- Miller, C., & Jezewski, M. A. (2001). A phenomenologic assessment of relapsing MS patients' experiences during treatment with interferon beta-1a. *Journal of Neuroscience Nursing, 33,* 240–244.
- Zahlis, E. H. (2001). The child's worries about the mother's breast cancer: Sources of distress in school-age children. *Oncology Nursing Forum, 28,* 1019–1025.

E. Special Projects

1. Suppose that you were interested in studying risky behavior among high school students. Describe how you might select a sample for your study using the following:

   a. A convenience sample
   b. A quota sample
   c. A cluster sample

2. Suppose you were interested in doing an in-depth study of the process of decision making regarding condom use among single men and women. Describe how you might select a sample for your study using the following:

   a. A maximum variation sample
   b. A homogeneous sample
   c. An extreme case sample
   d. A typical case sampling

3. Propose a researchable problem statement for a quantitative study. Specify a research and sampling design to study this problem. In particular, specify the following:

   a. The target population
   b. An accessible population
   c. Specific eligibility criteria for sampling
   d. A sampling design, together with a rationale
   e. A recommended sample size

   With respect to the latter three aspects, be realistic. Take into account your resources, time, and level of expertise. That is, recommend a plan that would be feasible to implement.

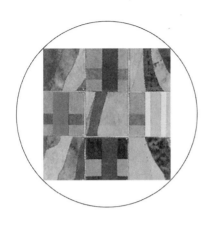

PART 4

Measurement and Data Collection

CHAPTER **14**

Designing and Implementing a Data Collection Plan

A. Matching Exercises

Match each descriptive statement regarding data collection methods from Set B with one (or more) of the statements from Set A. Indicate the letter(s) corresponding to your response next to each item in Set B.

SET A
a. Self-reports
b. Observations
c. Biophysiologic measures
d. None of the above

SET B	**RESPONSE**
1. Cannot easily be gathered unobtrusively	_____
2. Can be biased by the subject's desire to "look good"	_____
3. Can be used to gather data from infants	_____
4. Is rarely used in qualitative studies	_____
5. Is a good way to obtain information about human *behavior*	_____
6. Can be biased by the researcher's values and beliefs	_____
7. Can be combined with other data collection methods in a single study	_____
8. Can range from highly unstructured to highly structured data	_____
9. Can yield quantitative information	_____
10. Benefits from pretesting	_____

B. Completion Exercises

Write the words or phrases that correctly complete the following sentences.

1. The four dimensions along which data collection methods can vary are

   _____, _____, _____, and

   _____ .

2. _____ is the dimension that could result in distortions on the part
   of subjects who are engaged in socially unacceptable behavior.

3. The data collection approach that is especially high on objectivity is

   _____ .

4. When we want to know what people's attitudes are, we are most likely to use
   the method of _____ .

5. Nonverbal communication would most likely be studied using the method of

   _____ .

6. When quantitative data are used qualitatively, the process is referred to as
   _____ the data.

7. In a quantitative study, the first step is usually to create an inventory of

   _____ .

8. When a researcher analyzes outcomes for subsets of the sample, this is called
   a search for _____ .

9. Researchers sometimes collect data to conduct a(n) _____, to
   determine if an intervention was actually implemented as planned.

10. In selecting an existing instrument for use in a study, the primary consideration
    is _____ .

11. If the population has literacy problems, it may be important to assess a self-
    report instrument for its _____ .

12. If an instrument is copyrighted, it is necessary to obtain
    _____ before it can be used.

13. An instrument package should be _____ to determine the
    amount of time it takes to collect the data.

14. Data collection _____ spell out the specific procedures to be used in collecting the data.

15. When interview data are collected in person by an interviewer reading questions from and entering data onto a computer, the procedure is called _____.

16. The qualitative research tradition that typically collects a wide array of data from a variety of sources is _____.

17. To ensure that qualitative data are the verbatim responses of participants, interviews should be _____ and then later _____.

18. When qualitative researchers get overly involved with their participants, they commit the pitfall that is called _____.

C. Study Questions

1. Define the following terms. Compare your definition with the definition in Chapter 14 or in the glossary of the textbook.

   a. Data collection plan: _____

   _____

   b. Records: _____

   _____

   c. Instrument:_____

   _____

   d. Objectivity:_____

   _____

   e. Self-report: _____

   _____

   f. Observer bias: _____

   _____

g. Norms: _____

_____

h. Training manual: _____

_____

i. Audio-CASI: _____

_____

j. Reflexivity: _____

_____

2. Below are several research problems. Indicate what methods of data collection (self-report, observation, biophysiologic measures) you might recommend using for each. Defend your response.

a. How does an elderly patient manage the transition from hospital to home?

_____

b. What are the predictors of intravenous site symptoms?

_____

c. What are the factors associated with smoking during pregnancy?

_____

d. To what extent and in what manner do nurses interact differently with male and female patients?

_____

e. What are the coping mechanisms of parents whose infants are long-term patients in neonatal intensive care units?

_____

3. For each of the research problems in Question C.2, indicate where on the four dimensions discussed in this chapter (structure, quantifiability, researcher obtrusiveness, and objectivity) the method of data collection would most likely lie.

4. Read the following article and describe the data collection procedures in terms of the four dimensions discussed in this chapter:

Story, M., Lytle, L. A., Birnbaum, A. S., & Perry, C. L. (2002). Peer-led, school-based nutrition education for young adolescents: Feasibility and process evaluation of the TEENS study. *Journal of School Health, 72,* 121–127.

5. Read the following article, which relied exclusively on self-report, and identify variables that *could* have been measured with an alternative approach:

Dormire, S. L., & Yarandi, H. (2001). Predictors of risk for adolescent childbearing. *Applied Nursing Research, 14*, 81–86.

D. Application Exercises

1. Here is a brief summary of a fictitious study. Read the summary and then respond to the questions that follow.

   Crampton (2003) was interested in studying a variety of psychological effects (e.g., stress, self-esteem, depression, body image) among women who give birth by cesarean delivery. She designed a prospective study that allowed her to compare three groups of primiparas: women who gave birth vaginally, those who had a planned cesarean delivery, and those who had an emergency cesarean delivery. According to the research design, data were to be collected in the sixth month of the pregnancy and then again 2 weeks after delivery.

   When Crampton began to make a list of the variables she wanted to measure, she realized that the data collection would require a considerable amount of time, particularly with respect to the measurement of the dependent variables. Given that levels of pain, fatigue, and preoccupation were expected to be high in the postpartum period, she decided to focus on a single psychological outcome, namely depression.

   Crampton developed three instrument packages: one for administration during the subjects' pregnancies, a second for administration postpartum, and a third consisting of forms for the extraction of information from medical and hospital records. The variables to be measured in each included the following:

   1. *Predelivery self-report.* Demographic information (e.g., age, marital status, employment status and occupation, educational background); pregnancy history; attitudes toward and expectations about cesarean delivery; level of depression
   2. *Postpartum self-report.* Updated background information (e.g., expected date of return to work, if applicable); perception of the birth experience; levels of fatigue and pain; level of depression
   3. *Medical information.* Weight gain during pregnancy; prenatal history (e.g., number of prenatal visits, use of vitamins, sonogram history); method of delivery and reason for cesarean, if applicable; gestational length; infant status (e.g., birth weight, length, Apgar score)

   Based on a colleague's recommendation, Crampton decided to use the Center for Epidemiological Studies Depression (CES-D) Scale as her main dependent variable. She developed all other questions herself. Crampton pretested the predelivery self-report instruments with 10 pregnant women and the postpartum instruments with 10 women who had recently delivered, five of whom had had a cesarean delivery. Crampton used a nurse assistant to help her collect the data. The assistant had helped her prepare the instruments, so no formal training was thought to be needed.

   Review and critique the description of the overall study. Suggest possible alternative ways of collecting the data for the research problem. To assist you in your critique, here are some guiding questions:

a. Most of the data in this study were collected by self-report. Could the data have been collected in another way? *Should* they have been, in your opinion?

b. Comment on the degree of structure of the instruments used. Would you recommend more structured or less structured instruments? Why or why not?

c. Comment on the researcher's overall data collection decisions and approach to developing the instrument package.

d. Were the instruments adequately pretested?

e. Comment on the researcher's method of actually collecting the data, including the use of other personnel.

2. Below are several suggested research articles. Skim one or more of these articles, paying particular attention to the methods used to measure research variables and collect the data. Then respond to questions a through e from Question D.1 in terms of this actual research study, to the extent possible.

- Hendrich, A. L., Bender, P. S., & Nyhuis, A. (2003). Validation of the Hendrich II Fall Risk Model: A large concurrent case/control study of hospitalized patients. *Applied Nursing Research, 16,* 9–21.
- Kishida, Y. (2001). Anxiety in Japanese women after elective abortion. *Journal of Obstetric, Gynecologic, and Neonatal Nursing, 30,* 490–495.
- McDonald, D. D., & Weiskopf, C. S. (2001). Adult patients' postoperative pain descriptions and responses to the Short Form McGill Pain Questionnaire. *Clinical Nursing Research, 10,* 442–452.
- Salazar, M. K., Kemerer, S., Amman, M. C., & Fabrey, L. J. (2002). Defining the roles and functions of occupational and environmental health nurses: Results of a national job analysis. *AAOHN Journal, 50,* 16–25.
- Stover, J. C., Skelly, A. H., Holditch-Davis, D., & Dunn, P. F. (2001). Perceptions of health and their relationship to symptoms in African American women with Type 2 diabetes. *Applied Nursing Research, 14,* 72–80.

3. Below are several suggested qualitative research articles. Skim one or more of these articles, paying particular attention to the methods used to collect the data. Then respond to the following questions in terms of this actual research study, to the extent possible.

a. What types of data were collected?

b. Where on the four dimensions of data collection do the data lie?

c. How were data recorded and stored?

d. What special fieldwork issues (if any) arose during the course of data collection?

- Boutain, D. M. (2001). Discourses of worry, stress, and high blood pressure in rural south Louisiana. *Journal of Nursing Scholarship, 33,* 225–230.
- Hurst, I. (2001). Vigilant watching over: Mothers' actions to safeguard their premature babies in the newborn intensive care nursery. *Journal of Perinatal & Neonatal Nursing, 15,* 39–57.

- Labun, E. (2001). Cultural discovery in nursing practice with Vietnamese clients. *Journal of Advanced Nursing, 35,* 874–881.
- Mahoney, J. S. (2001). An ethnographic approach to understanding the illness experiences of patients with congestive heart failure and their family members. *Heart & Lung, 30,* 429–436.
- Wilde, M. H. (2002). Urine flowing: A phenomenological study of living with a urinary catheter. *Research in Nursing & Health , 25,* 14–24.

E. Special Projects

1. Read one of the studies suggested in Question D.2. Based on this study, write the Background section (Section I.A. in Table 14-1 of the textbook) for a training manual for this study.

2. Suppose you wanted to do an ethnographic study of the culture of a public health clinic adjacent to an urban public housing project. What types of data would you collect? How might you record and store your data? How might you go about gaining the trust of clients and of staff and volunteers?

CHAPTER **15**

Collecting Self-Report Data

A. Matching Exercises

1. Match each descriptive statement regarding self-report methods from Set B with one of the statements from Set A. Indicate the letter corresponding to your response next to each item in Set B.

SET A
a. Interviews
b. Questionnaires
c. Both interviews and questionnaires
d. Neither interviews nor questionnaires

SET B   **RESPONSE**

1. Can provide respondents the protection of anonymity   _____

2. Can be used with illiterate respondents   _____

3. Can contain both open- and closed-ended questions   _____

4. Is used in grounded theory studies   _____

5. Is the best way to measure human behavior   _____

6. Generally yields high response rates   _____

7. Can control the order in which questions are asked and
   answered   _____

8. Is generally an inexpensive method of data collection   _____

9. Requires that the purpose of the study be unknown to the
   study participant   _____

10. Benefits from pretesting   _____

11. Can be used in longitudinal studies   _____

12. Can be distributed by mail   _____

2. Match each descriptive statement from Set B with one of the statements from Set A. Indicate the letter corresponding to your response next to each item in Set B.

SET A

a. Likert scales
b. Semantic differential scales
c. Both Likert and semantic differential scales
d. Neither Likert nor semantic differential scales

SET B	**RESPONSE**
1. Permits fine discriminations among respondents	_____
2. Can be used to measure attitudes	_____
3. Is sometimes referred to as a summated rating scale	_____
4. Is subject to response-set biases	_____
5. Is often used to measure behavioral characteristics	_____
6. Presents statements to which respondents indicate agreement or disagreement	_____
7. Rarely contains more than five items	_____
8. Can yield an evaluation, activity, and potency dimension	_____
9. Uses item reversals to minimize response-set biases such as acquiescence	_____
10. Provides a quantitative measure of an attribute	_____

B. Completion Exercises

Write the words or phrase s that correctly complete the following sentences.

1. Completely unstructured interviews generally begin with a broad, informal question, sometimes referred to as a _____ question.

2. In ethnographic interviews, researchers might ask _____, _____, and _____ questions.

3. In semistructured interviews, general question areas are normally listed on a(n) _____.

4. When a group of respondents is assembled in one place to discuss questions simultaneously, the interview is called a(n) _____ .

5. Ethnographers sometimes use _____ (narratives about people's life experiences) as a way to learn about cultural patterns.

6. The approach used to question people about key events, decisions, or turning points is referred to as the _____ technique.

7. The _____ method is used to gather information about cognitive processes, such as decision making.

8. A disadvantage of _____ questions is that researchers may inadvertently omit some potentially important response alternatives.

9. _____ questions are relatively inefficient in terms of the respondents' time.

10. If respondents are not very verbal or articulate, _____ questions are generally most appropriate.

11. The type of instrument that typically uses more closed-ended than open-ended questions is the _____ .

12. Questions that offer only two response options are known as _____ items.

13. Another term for two-dimensional checklists is _____ .

14. Likert scales consist of a number of statements written in the _____ form.

15. Some people omit the category labeled _____ in constructing Likert scales, to avoid "fence-sitting."

16. In Likert scales, positively worded statements are scored in one direction, and the scoring of negatively worded statements is _____ .

17. Respondents rate concepts on a series of bipolar adjectives in the _____ technique.

18. Interviewer probes should always be _____ .

19. Respondents are less likely to give "don't know" responses in a(n) _____ situation than on a questionnaire.

20. Nonresponse in self-report studies is generally not _____ and can therefore lead to bias.

21. The bias introduced when respondents select options at either end of the response continuum is known as _____ .

22. Response alternatives should be mutually _____ .

C. Study Questions

1. Define the following terms. Compare your definition with the definition in Chapter 15 or in the glossary of the textbook.

   a. Unstructured interview: _____

   _____

   b. Focus group moderator: _____

   _____

   c. Joint interview: _____

   _____

   d. Oral history:_____

   _____

   e. Photo elicitation:_____

   _____

   f. Interview schedule: _____

   _____

   g. Questionnaire:_____

   _____

   h. Open-ended question: _____

   _____

   i. Fixed-alternative question:_____

   _____

   j. Cover letter:_____

   _____

   k. Rating question: _____

   _____

l. Visual analogue scale: _____

_____

m. Social psychological scale:_____

_____

n. Module: _____

_____

o. Follow-up reminder:_____

_____

p. Probe:_____

_____

q. Response rate:_____

_____

r. Response set:_____

_____

s. Social desirability response set: _____

_____

t. Acquiescence response set:_____

_____

u. Nay-sayer: _____

_____

2. Below are several research problems. Indicate which type of unstructured approach you might recommend using for each. Defend your response.

   a. By what process do parents of a handicapped child learn to cope with their child's disability?

   _____

   _____

   b. What are the barriers to preventive health care practices among the urban poor?

   _____

   _____

c. What stresses does the spouse of a terminally ill patient experience?

_____

_____

d. What type of information does a nurse draw on most heavily in formulating nursing diagnoses?

_____

_____

e. What are the coping mechanisms and perceived barriers to coping among severely disfigured burn patients?

_____

_____

3. Suppose you were interested in studying the frustrations of patients waiting for treatment in the waiting area of an emergency department. Develop a topic guide for a focused interview on this topic.

4. For the study described in Question C.3, develop 10 closed-ended questions. Compare the nature of the information you would obtain for the research problem described in Question C.3 using the topic guide versus using the closed-ended questions. Which approach would yield more useful information? Defend your response.

5. Suppose you were interested in studying risky behavior among adolescents. Develop the following types of questions designed to measure these behaviors.

a. Dichotomous item
b. Multiple choice item
c. Open-ended item

6. Below are hypothetical responses for Respondent Y and Respondent Z to the Likert statements presented in Table 15-2 of the textbook. What would the total score for both of these respondents be, using the scoring rules described in Chapter 15?

Item No.	Respondent Y	Respondent Z
1	D	SA
2	A	D
3	SA	D
4	?	A
5	D	SA
6	SA	D
Total score:	____	____

7. Below are hypothetical responses for Respondents A, B, C, and D to the Likert statements presented in Table 15-2 of the text. Three of these four sets of responses contain some indication of a possible response-set bias. Identify *which* three, and identify the types of bias.

Item No.	Respondent A	Respondent B	Respondent C	Respondent D
1	A	SA	SD	D
2	A	SD	SA	SD
3	SA	D	SA	D
4	A	A	SD	SD
5	SA	A	SD	SD
6	SA	SD	SA	D
Bias:	___	___	___	___

8. Below are 10 attitudinal statements regarding attitudes toward natural family planning. For each statement, indicate how you think the item would be scored (i.e., would "strongly agree" be assigned a score of 1 or 5, assuming high scores reflect more favorable attitudes?). What are the maximum and minimum scores possible on this scale?

Maximum score: _____; minimum score: _____

STATEMENT	SCORE FOR "STRONGLY AGREE"
a. Natural family planning is an effective method of avoiding unwanted pregnancies.	___
b. Natural family planning removes the spontaneity from lovemaking.	___
c. Using natural family planning methods is too time-consuming.	___
d. A man and a woman can be drawn closer together by collaborating on using natural family planning.	___
e. Natural family planning is the safest form of birth control.	___
f. Natural family planning is too risky if you really don't want a pregnancy.	___
g. Natural family planning puts a woman in better touch with her body.	___
h. Natural family planning is an acceptable form of contraception.	___
i. All in all, natural family planning is the best method of birth control.	___
j. Natural family planning is "unnatural" in terms of the restrictions it imposes on lovemaking.	___

9. Identify five constructs of clinical relevance that would be appropriate for measurement using a visual analogue scale (VAS).

10. Suggest response alternatives for the following questions that might appear in a questionnaire.

   a. In a typical month, how frequently do you practice breast self-examination?

   _____

   b. When was the last time you had your blood pressure tested?

   _____

   c. Which of the following statements best describes your attitude toward nurse practitioners?

   _____

   d. What is your marital status?

   _____

   e. How would you rate your nursing research instruction in terms of overall quality of teaching?

   _____

   f. How often do you skip breakfast?

   _____

   g. How important is it to you to avoid a pregnancy at this time?

   _____

   h. How many cigarettes do you smoke in a typical day?

   _____

   i. From which of the following sources have you learned about the dangers of smoking?

   _____

   j. Which of the following statements best describes the physical pain you experienced during labor and delivery?

   _____

D. Application Exercises

1. Here is a brief summary of a fictitious study. Read the summary and then respond to the questions that follow.

   Kane (2003) conducted a survey that focused on drug use patterns in an urban adolescent population. The survey used self-administered questionnaires that were distributed to 25 high schools and administered in group (homeroom) sessions to 3568 respondents. The questionnaire consisted of 56 closed-ended and 2 open-ended questions. Included were background questions; questions on the students' attitudes toward, knowledge of, and experience with various drugs; and questions on the students' physical and mental health. The instrument was pretested with 10 college freshmen before administration.

Review and critique the above description of the overall study. Suggest possible alternative ways of collecting the data for the research problem. To assist you in your critique, here are some guiding questions:

a. The data in this study were collected by self-report. Could the data have been collected in another way? *Should* they have been, in your opinion?

b. Were the data collected by questionnaire or interview? Was the decision to use this method appropriate, or would you recommend an alternative procedure? Comment on the advantages and disadvantages of the procedure used for this particular research problem.

c. Comment on the degree of structure of the instrument used. Would you recommend a more structured or a less structured instrument? Why or why not?

d. Was the instrument adequately pretested?

e. Comment on the methods by which the instrument was administered. Were the methods efficient? Did they yield an adequate response rate? Did they appear costly? What opportunity did respondents have to obtain clarifying information about the questions?

2. Below are several suggested research articles. Skim one or more of these articles, paying particular attention to the methods used to collect the self-report data. Then respond to questions a through e from Question D.1 in terms of this actual research study.

- Bialoskurski, M. M., Cox, C. L., Wiggins, R. D. (2002). The relationship between maternal needs and priorities in a neonatal intensive care environment. *Journal of Advanced Nursing, 37,* 62–69.
- Davis, T., Ross, C., & MacDonald, G. F. (2002). Screening and assessing asthmatics for anxiety disorders. *Clinical Nursing Research, 11,* 173–189.
- Eller, L. S. (2001). Quality of life in persons living with HIV. *Clinical Nursing Research, 10,* 401–423.
- Ip, W., Chau, J., Change, A., & Liu, M. (2001). Knowledge of and attitudes toward sex among Chinese adolescents. *Western Journal of Nursing Research, 23,* 211–222.
- Renker, P. R. (2002). "Keep A Blank Face. I Need To Tell You What Has Been Happening To Me." Teens' stories of abuse and violence before and during pregnancy. *MCN: The American Journal of Maternal/Child Nursing, 27,* 109–116.

3. Kane, in her study of drug use patterns among high school students, accompanied each questionnaire with the following cover letter:

Dear Student:

This questionnaire is part of a study to learn about some health-related issues among high school students. Through this study we hope to have a better understanding of young people in America. Students from 25 high schools in the United States are being asked to help us in this effort. Your high school was selected at random.

Your responses to this questionnaire are completely anonymous. No one will know your answers. So, even though some of the questions are very personal, we hope that you will answer honestly. The quality of the picture we will have of high school students today depends on your willingness to provide thorough and honest answers.

Please answer every question. When you are through, please turn the questionnaire in to your homeroom teacher.

Your cooperation in completing this questionnaire is deeply appreciated.

Sincerely,
Sarah Kane, R.N.

Review and critique this sample cover letter. Analyze the tone, wording, and content of the letter. Compare the content with the suggested contents of such a letter presented in Chapter 15 of the textbook.

4. Another brief summary of a fictitious study is presented next. Read the summary and then respond to the questions that follow.

   Thayer (2002) wanted to conduct a survey of nurses' attitudes toward abortion. For this study, she prepared 20 statements pro and con. After developing the items, she asked 10 of her colleagues to indicate their level of agreement or disagreement with the statements, on a seven-point scale. Thayer used the data from these 10 nurses as pretest data for refining the instrument. The original 20 items are presented below:
   1. Every woman has a right to obtain an abortion if she does not want a baby.
   2. Abortion should be made available to women on demand.
   *3. The government should subsidize the cost of abortions for poor women.
   4. Abortions should be made illegal.
   5. The right to an abortion should be available to all women.
   *6. Women whose lives are in danger because of their pregnancy should be allowed to have an abortion.
   7. Abortion is morally wrong.
   8. Women need to have control of their own bodies by having abortion services available to them.
   9. Women who have abortions are murderers.
   10. People who oppose abortions have no compassion for women's circumstances.
   11. Legalizing abortion is a sign of the decay of civilization.
   12. No decent woman would even consider killing her own baby through abortion.
   13. The freedom to choose an abortion is essential to the liberation of women.
   14. An enlightened society gives its citizens the right to make important choices, such as the decision to bear a child.
   15. The right to obtain a legal abortion should never be denied to women.
   16. Women who have abortions demonstrate the courage to make a tough decision.
   17. No woman should be forced to bear a baby she does not want.

*18. If men had to bear babies, abortions would never have been illegal.
19. Abortion is one of the most despicable acts that a human can commit.
20. Women should have the right to choose having an abortion.

Upon reviewing the pretest responses, Thayer eliminated items 3, 6, and 18 (indicated with an asterisk). She then had a 17-item scale ready to use in her survey.

Read and critique the description of Thayer's activities. Suggest possible alternative ways of collecting the data for the research problem. To assist you in your critique, here are some guiding questions:

   a. What type of scale did the researcher develop? Was this type of scale best suited to the researcher's needs, or would another type have been more appropriate? Why or why not?
   b. Given the researcher's aims, was the development of *any* type of scale appropriate? That is, could the data have been collected by another method? *Should* they have been, in your opinion?
   c. Comment on the procedures the researcher used to develop the scale. Was the scale adequately reviewed and pretested?
   d. Critique the quality of the scale itself. Does it consist of a sufficient number of items? Is the number of response alternatives good? Does the scale do an adequate job of minimizing bias? If not, suggest modifications that might reduce response-set biases.
   e. Do you think the scale is unidimensional? That is, does it appear to be measuring one (and only one) underlying concept?
   f. Comment on why you think the items that were eliminated (items 3, 6, and 18) were removed from the final scale.
   g. Do you feel the researcher needed to develop this scale from scratch?

5. Another brief summary of a fictitious study is presented next. Read the summary and then respond to the questions that follow.

   Kettlewell (2002) undertook an in-depth study of parents' experiences caring for children dying of cancer. The project was designed to describe the evolution of parents' caring practices in response to the demands of living with a dying child. Kettlewell conducted totally unstructured in-home interviews with one or both parents separately, beginning with the grand tour question, "Tell me about what happened when you first learned that your child was ill." Subsequently, Kettlewell conducted a more focused interview with both parents together (in homes where there were two parents). All interviews were tape recorded and later transcribed for analysis.

   a. The data in this study were collected through in-depth interview. Could the data have been collected in another way? *Should* it have been, in your opinion?
   b. Was the amount of structure in the data collection appropriate, or should there have been more or less structure?
   c. Comment on the method in which the data were collected (e.g., the setting, the use of tape recorders).

6. Below are several suggested research articles. Skim one or more of these articles, paying particular attention to the methods used to collect the self-report data. Respond to questions a through c from Question D.1 in terms of this actual research study.

- Ensign, J., & Panke, A. (2002). Barriers and bridges to care: voices of homeless female adolescent youth in Seattle, Washington, USA. *Journal of Advanced Nursing, 37,* 166–172.
- Kee, C. C., & Epps, C. D. (2001). Pain management practices of nurses caring for older patients with osteoarthritis. *Western Journal of Nursing Research, 23,* 195–210.
- Radley, A., & Taylor, D. (2003). Images of recovery: A photoelicitation study on the hospital ward. *Qualitative Health Research, 13,* 77–99.
- Shieh, C., & Kravitz, M. (2002). Maternal-fetal attachment in pregnant women who use illicit drugs. *Journal of Obstetric, Gynecologic, and Neonatal Nursing, 31,* 156–164.
- Wallace, D. C., Tuck, I., Boland, C. S., & Witucki, J. M. (2002). Client perceptions of parish nursing. *Public Health Nursing, 19,* 128–135.

E. Special Projects

1. Develop a short (2–3 pages) questionnaire, properly formatted and sequenced, for a study of pregnant women's attitudes toward breastfeeding.

2. Draft a cover letter to accompany the instrument developed in Exercise E.1.

3. Develop a topic guide that focuses on nursing students' reasons for selecting nursing as a career and their satisfactions and dissatisfactions with their decision. Administer the topic guide to five first-year nursing students in a face-to-face interview situation. Now administer the topic guide in a focus group setting with five nursing students. Compare the kinds of information that the two approaches yielded. What, if anything, did you learn in the group setting that did not emerge in the personal interviews (and vice versa)?

4. Develop semantic differential scales (i.e., a set of bipolar adjectives) to measure attitudes toward the following concepts: cancer, heart attack, AIDS, and brain damage.

5. Describe a potential use for the semantic differential scales described in Exercise E.4. What kinds of comparison might you make in such a study?

6. Construct a VAS to measure fatigue. Administer the VAS two ways: (1) to yourself at 10 different times of the day; and (2) to 10 different people at the same time of day. For the two types of administrations, is there similarity in scores, or is there a wide range of responses? Which of the two yields scores with a wider range?

CHAPTER **16**

Collecting Observational Data

A. Matching Exercises

Match each problem statement from Set B with one of the statements from Set A. Indicate the letter corresponding to your response next to each item in Set B.

SET A
a. The study would *require* observational data.
b. The study *could* use observational data as well as other forms of data.
c. The study is not amenable to observational data collection.

SET B   **RESPONSE**

1. Are nurses' attitudes toward abortion related to their years of nursing experience?   _____

2. Are patients' levels of stress related to their willingness to disclose their own fears to nursing staff?   _____

3. Are the sleep-wake patterns of infants related to their gestational age at birth?   _____

4. Is the degree of physical activity of a psychiatric patient related to his or her length of hospitalization?   _____

5. Are nurses' scores on a spiritual well-being scale related to their degree of comfort in instituting spiritual nursing interventions?   _____

6. Is a child's fear during immunization related to the nurse's method of preparing the child for the shot?   _____

7. Does the presence and behavior of a father in the delivery room affect a mother's level of pain?   _____

8. Is the ability of dialysis patients to cleanse and dress their shunts related to their self-esteem and locus of control?   _____

9. Is the level of achievement motivation among nursing students related to their clinical specialty?   _____

10. Is aggressive behavior among hospitalized mentally retarded children related to styles of discipline by hospital staff?   _____

B. Completion Exercises

Write the words or phrases that correctly complete the following sentences.

1. The major focus of observation in nursing research is the _____ and _____ of humans.

2. When the unit of observation is small, specific behaviors, the approach is said to be _____ .

3. The reactive measurement effect may occur when the observer is not_____ .

4. If a researcher used a directed setting, the study would be high on the _____ dimension.

5. The technique known as _____ involves the collection of unstructured observational data in which observers play a role in the group or culture being observed.

6. The fourth phase of a participant observer's role involves _____ _____ .

7. The most highly focused type of observation, according to Spradley's method, is _____ observation.

8. The three major types of observational positioning in participant observation studies are _____, _____, and _____ positioning.

9. Chronologic notes about observers' use of their time are maintained in a(n)_____.

10. The three types of reflective field notes are _____,
    _____, and _____notes.

11. In structured observations, the most common procedure is to construct a(n)
    _____ that designates the behaviors or events to be
    observed.

12. In general, less observer inference is required when the units of behavior being
    observed are _____ .

13. Checklists for nonexhaustive systems are sometimes referred to as (n)
    _____.

14. _____ is the method of obtaining representative observations
    by selecting time periods during which observations will occur.

15. Observers need to be carefully _____ in the use of a structured
    observational instrument.

16. The tendency for observers to rate things too positively is a bias known as the
    _____ .

17. An observer bias in which extreme events are given mid-range ratings is known
    as a bias toward _____ .

18. The tendency for observers to rate things too negatively is a bias known as the
    _____ .

C. Study Questions

1. Define the following terms. Compare your definition with the definition in
   Chapter 16 or in the glossary of the textbook.

   a. Molar unit of analysis: _____

   _____

   b. Reactivity: _____

   _____

   c. Directed setting: _____

   _____

    d. Windshield survey: _____

_____

    e. Descriptive observations: _____

_____

    f. Multiple positioning: _____

_____

    g. Mobile positioning: _____

_____

    h. Field notes: _____

_____

    i. Jottings: _____

_____

    j. Checklist: _____

_____

    k. Rating scale: _____

_____

    l. Event sampling: _____

_____

    m. Central tendency bias: _____

_____

    n. Enhancement of contrast bias: _____

_____

    o. Halo effect: _____

_____

2. Below are several problem statements in which the dependent variable is amenable to observation. Indicate your recommendation for the relationship between the observer and study participants along the concealment and intervention dimensions for each problem. Justify your response.

    a. What is the effect of touch on the crying behavior of hospitalized children?

_____

_____

b. What is the effect of increased patient/staff ratios in psychiatric hospitals on interpersonal conflict among patients?

_____

_____

c. Does a patient's need for personal space vary as a function of age?

_____

_____

d. Are the self-grooming activities of nursing home patients related to the frequency of visits from friends and relatives?

_____

_____

e. What is the process by which very-low-birth-weight infants develop the sucking response?

_____

_____

f. What type of patient behaviors are most likely to elicit empathic behaviors in nurses?

_____

_____

g. Do nurses reinforce passive behaviors among female patients more than among male patients?

_____

_____

3. For each of the problem statements indicated above in Exercise C.2, specify whether you think a structured or unstructured approach would be preferable. Justify your response.

a. _____

_____

b. _____

_____

c. _____

_____

d. _____

_____

e. _____

_____

f. _____

_____

g. _____

_____

4. Suppose that you were interested in studying verbal interactions among nursing faculty with respect to expressions of solidarity versus antagonism. Would you recommend a molecular unit of analysis (e.g., individual words) or a more molar unit of analysis (e.g., sentences or entire dialogues from staff meetings)? Justify your response.

D. Application Exercises

1. A brief summary of a fictitious observational study follows. Read the summary and then respond to the questions that follow.

Nolte (2003) studied hospitalized patients' requests for nursing assistance in relation to their age, gender, and number of daily outside visitors. Her central hypothesis was that patient requests were higher among those with few or no visitors. Subjects for the study were 100 patients on a medical-surgical unit of a 500-bed hospital in New Jersey. All 100 subjects were patients admitted for relatively routine procedures, such as appendectomies; none was terminally ill. Observations were made by the nursing staff, who were instructed to record verbatim all requests that subjects made during a 24-hour period and all instances of patients' use of the call button. At the end of each shift, each nurse rated the patient on seven-point scales along several dimensions, such as talkative/not talkative, hostile/friendly, and in no pain/in great pain.

Each request for assistance was categorized according to a system that Nolte had developed. The categories included requests in the following areas: medication; food or beverage; environmental change (e.g., temperature or light adjustment); physician consultation; reading material, television, or radio; assistance (e.g., getting in/out of bed); and conversation or emotional support. Nolte performed all of the categorizations herself based on the nurses' verbatim accounts. Nolte found that the number of patients' requests was unrelated to their gender and age, although there were age and gender differences in the types of requests made. Patients with no visitors made significantly more requests than patients with one or more visitors on the day of the observation, and patients with no visitors were also somewhat more likely to be rated as unfriendly.

Review and critique this study. Suggest alternative ways of collecting the data for the research problem. To assist you in your critique, here are some guiding questions:

 a. The data in this study were collected by observation. Could the data have been collected in another way? *Should* they have been, in your opinion?
 b. Specify the relationship between the observer and those being observed on the concealment and intervention dimensions. Do you feel that the specified relationship is appropriate? What kinds of problems might it raise?
 c. In terms of the unit of observation, would you describe the approach as basically molar or molecular? Do you think that the level of observation is appropriate, or would you recommend an approach that is more molar or more molecular?
 d. Would you classify the study as having used an unstructured or structured observational procedure? Was the amount of structure in the data collection appropriate, or should there have been more or less structure?
 e. Was the specific procedure used to capture the study variables an adequate way to operationalize the variables? Could you recommend any improvements?
 f. What type of sampling plan was used to sample observations in this study? Would an alternative sampling plan have been better? Why or why not?
 g. What types of observational bias do you think might be operational in this study?
 h. Comment on the appropriateness of the individuals who made the observations. Can you identify any potential problems with respect to the internal and external validity of the study?

2. Below are several suggested research articles in which a structured observational approach was used. Review one of the articles and respond to questions a through h from Question D.1, to the extent possible, in terms of this study.

 • Drevenhorn, E., Håkansson, A., & Petersson, K. (2001). Counseling hypertensive patients. *Clinical Nursing Research, 10,* 369–386.
 • Kovach, C. R., & Wells, T. (2002). Pacing of activity as a predictor of agitation for persons with dementia in acute care. *Journal of Gerontological Nursing, 28,* 28–35.
 • Modrcin-Talbott, M. A., Harrison, L. L., Groer, M. W., & Younger, M. S. (2003). The biobehavioral effects of gentle human touch on preterm infants. *Nursing Science Quarterly, 16,* 60–67.
 • Pressler, J. L., & Hepworth, J. T. (2002). A quantitative use of the NIDCAP tool. *Clinical Nursing Research, 11,* 89–102.
 • Symanski, M. E., Hayes, M. J., & Akilesh, M. K. (2002). Patterns of premature newborns' sleep-wake states before and after nursing interventions on the night shift. *Journal of Obstetric, Gynecologic, and Neonatal Nursing, 31,* 305–313.

3. A brief summary of another fictitious observational study follows. Read the summary and then respond to questions a to h from Question D.1., to the extent possible.

> Roberts (2003) studied the transitions of elderly people from an assisted living facility to a nursing home. Over the 3 months of summer, she volunteered at a 50-bed nursing home in the Midwest region of the United States. During this 3-month period, eight new residents were admitted to the nursing home from assisted living facilities. Each resident signed an informed consent explaining that they were agreeing to participate in a study of their adjustment to the nursing home. Roberts used participant observation to collect the data. Every Monday, Wednesday, and Friday from 8:00 AM to 4:00 PM, Roberts observed the nursing home residents' behavior and activities. She observed the admission interview of each of the eight new elders to the nursing home. She participated in the nursing home activities with the residents (e.g., bingo, meals, crafts). Roberts periodically interviewed not only the elders about their feelings and experiences making the transition, but also their family members who visited the elders. She kept a daily journal of her fieldwork at the nursing home. In addition, she created a daily checklist she used to chart the different activities of the nursing home residents in her sample and the length of time they participated in each activity.

4. Below are several suggested research articles in which an unstructured observational approach was used. Review one of the articles and respond to questions a through h from Question D.1, to the extent possible, in terms of this study.

- Clark, L. (2002). Mexican-origin mothers' experiences using children's health care services. *Western Journal of Nursing Research, 24,* 159–179.
- Costello, J. (2001). Nursing older dying patients: Findings from an ethnographic study of death and dying in elderly care wards. *Journal of Advanced Nursing, 35,* 59–68.
- Domian, E. W. (2001). Cultural practices and social support of pregnant women in a northern New Mexico community. *Journal of Nursing Scholarship, 33,* 331–336.
- Pincharoen S., & Congdon, J. G. (2003). Spirituality and health in older Thai persons in the United States. *Western Journal of Nursing Research, 25,* 93–108
- Rutherford, M. S., & Roux, G. M. (2002). Health beliefs and practices in rural El Salvador: An ethnographic study. *Journal of Cultural Diversity, 9,* 3–11.

E. Special Projects

1. Below is a list of five variables. Indicate briefly how you would operationalize each using structured observational procedures.

   a. Fear in hospitalized children
   b. Pain during childbirth

    c. Dependency in psychiatric patients

    d. Empathy in nursing students

    e. Cooperativeness in chemotherapy patients

2. Develop five problem statements for studies that could be implemented using observational procedures.

3. Develop a problem statement for a study that would involve participant observation. Analyze the strengths and weaknesses of using this approach for your problem.

4. Suppose you wanted to study facial expressions in autistic children. Describe the sampling plan you would recommend for such a study.

CHAPTER **17**

Collecting Biophysiologic and Other Data

A. Matching Exercises

Match each descriptive statement regarding a data collection approach from Set B with one (or more) of the statements from Set A. Indicate the letter(s) corresponding to your response next to each item in Set B.

SET A
a. Biophysiologic measure
b. Vignette
c. Projective technique
d. Q sort
e. Records
f. Cognitive tests
g. None of the above

SET B   **RESPONSE**

1. May be subject to selective survival bias   _____

2. May require advanced training for interpretation _____

3. Does not depend on respondents' conscious cooperation to provide information about themselves   _____

4. Can measure behaviors and events   _____

5. Is susceptible to response set biases   _____

6. Can be used to measure personality characteristics _____

7. Can yield or involve qualitative data   _____

8. An IQ test is an example   _____

9. Is used in most nursing research studies   _____

10. Yields ipsative data   _____

11. Can be administered by mail   _____

12. Often involves complex instrumentation systems   _____

B. Completion Exercises

Write the words or phrases that correctly complete the following sentences.

1. Biophysiologic measures that are taken directly within a living organism are

   _____ measures.

2. The entire set of apparatus and equipment used in connection with biophysio-

   logic measurements is referred to as the _____ .

3. When biophysiologic materials are extracted from people and subjected to

   analysis, the data are referred to as _____ measures.

4. The major advantage of using existing records is that they are

   _____.

5. In a Q sort, subjects are generally instructed to place most of the cards near the

   _____ of the distribution.

6. In Q sorts, forcing subjects to place a predetermined number of cards in each

   pile helps eliminate _____ .

7. Because of its forced-choice nature, the Q-sort technique yields

   _____ measures.

8. The Thematic Apperception Test (TAT) is an example of the method of

   _____ projective techniques.

9. The projective technique in which subjects are presented with a verbal stimu-

   lus to which to respond is known as a(n) _____ technique.

10. _____ are brief descriptions of individuals or situations to

    which subjects are asked to react.

C. Study Questions

1. Define the following terms. Compare your definition with the definition in
   Chapter 17 or in the glossary of the textbook.

   a. Biophysiologic measure: _____

_____

   b. Instrumentation system: _____

_____

   c. Records: _____

_____

   d. Selective deposit bias: _____

_____

   e. Q sort: _____

_____

   f. Normative measures: _____

_____

   g. Projective techniques: _____

_____

   h. Sentence-completion technique:_____

_____

   i. Cognitive test: _____

_____

2. Below are five statements that might appear on Q-sort cards. For each, describe one or more continua according to which the cards could be sorted (e.g., one continuum could be "very much like me/not at all like me" for a statement such as, "I like to go to parties").

   a. Americans should change their diets. _____

   b. I am bothered by the uncertainty of my prognosis. _____

   c. Acid indigestion _____

   d. Nursing care during most recent hospitalization _____

   e. Freedom from pain _____

3. Indicate which of the measures below is an in vivo measure and which is an in vitro measure:

   a. Direct blood pressure measures_____

   b. Electrocardiogram measures _____

c. Hemoglobin concentration _____

d. Total lung capacity _____

e. Blood gas analysis of P_{CO_2} _____

f. Chronoscope measures _____

g. Nasopharyngeal culture _____

h. Goniometer readings _____

i. Palmar Sweat Index _____

j. Blood pH _____

4. Three nurse researchers were collaborating on a study of the effect of preoperative visits to surgical patients by operating room nurses on the stress levels of those patients just before surgery. One researcher wanted to use the patients' self-reports to measure stress; the second suggested using pulse rate and the Palmer Sweat Index; the third recommended using an observational measure of stress. Which measure do you think would be the most appropriate for this research problem? Can you suggest other possible measures of stress that might be even more appropriate? Justify your response.

5. Suppose you were interested in middle-aged people's reactions to the prospect of eventually living in a nursing home. Develop five incomplete sentences that could be used to obtain the information by the sentence-completion technique.

a. _____

b. _____

c. _____

d. _____

e. _____

6. Identify five types of available records readily accessible to nurses that could be used to conduct a research study, and indicate some variables available from those sources.

a. _____

b. _____

c. _____

d. _____

e. _____

7. What are some of the advantages and disadvantages of a Q sort, as compared with a Likert scale?
8. Below is a study in which vignettes were used. Can you suggest alternative methods of collecting the data? Would the alternative have been preferable in terms of the quality of data obtained?

> Early, M. R., & Williams, R. A. (2002). Emergency nurses' experience with violence: Does it affect nursing care of battered women? *Journal of Emergency Nursing, 28,* 199–204.

D. Application Exercises

1. A summary of a fictitious study is presented next. Read the summary and then respond to the questions that follow.

> Walbridge-Allen (2003) used a combination of projective techniques to study children's fears of hospitalization. Forty children were randomly assigned to an experimental or control condition. The experimental group received a special treatment designed to alleviate prehospitalization anxiety in school-aged children. Controls did not receive any special instruction or treatment. The groups were then compared in terms of their responses to several projective measures, including the following:
>
> • Responses to three cartoons that showed a hospitalized child interacting with hospital staff in three settings (as the child was being taken to the operating room, as the child was given medication, and as the child was eating). The children were asked to complete the dialogue by indicating the response of the hospitalized child.
> • Sentence completions that included the following stems:
>
> I think nurses are . . .
>
> Being in a hospital is . . .
>
> I feel . . .
>
> • Play technique involving the use of dolls. Two dolls are given to the child, and the child is asked to play out a scene between a hospitalized child and a playmate who comes to visit him or her in the hospital.

Read and critique the description of Walbridge-Allen's activities. Suggest possible alternative ways of collecting the data for the research problem. To assist you in your critique, here are some guiding questions:

  a. Which of the methods described in this chapter did the researcher employ? Was this a good selection? Would you recommend that the researcher switch to an alternative method, such as other methods described in Chapter 17, or methods discussed in Chapters 15 or 16? Why or why not?
  b. Comment on the techniques used in terms of response-set biases.
  c. Comment on the techniques used in terms of the degree of objectivity of measuring the critical variables.

d. Comment on the techniques used in terms of the efficiency of the procedure (i.e., amount of time required by subjects and researcher in relationship to the amount of data yielded).

e. Comment on the techniques used in terms of their appropriateness for the study sample.

2. Below are several suggested research articles in which a projective technique was used. Review one of the articles and respond to questions a through e from Question D.1, to the extent possible, in terms of this actual study.

- Carroll, M. K., & Ryan-Wenger, N. A. (1999). School-age children's fears, anxiety, and human figure drawings. *Journal of Pediatric Health Care, 13,* 24–31.
- Herth, K. (1998). Hope as seen through the eyes of homeless children. *Journal of Advanced Nursing, 28,* 1053–1062.
- Kennedy, C. M., & Rodriguez, D. A. (1999). Risk taking in young Hispanic children. *Journal of Pediatric Health Care, 13,* 126–135.
- Pradel, F. G., Hartzema, A.G., & Bush P. J. (2001). Asthma self-management: The perspective of children. *Patient Education & Counseling, 45,* 199–209.
- Sartain, S. A., Clarke, C. L., & Heyman, R. (2000). Hearing the voices of children with chronic illness. *Journal of Advanced Nursing, 32,* 913–921.

3. A summary of another fictitious study follows next. Read the summary and then respond to the questions that follow.

> Forester (2002) conducted a quasi-experimental study of the effectiveness of a program for treating the physiologic anemia associated with pregnancy. The experimental treatment involved instruction regarding a nutritional regimen. The experimental group received verbal instructions by a nurse-midwife regarding dietary requirements and a list of foods known to be high in iron. Recommended daily amounts of certain foods were prescribed. The intervention also involved follow-up telephone conversations with the experimental group members at the 30th and 34th weeks of the pregnancy to discuss dietary and nutritional concerns. The comparison group members were given information that is normally given to pregnant women, with no individual follow-up. Fifty pregnant women who were outpatients at one hospital clinic served as experimental subjects, and 50 pregnant women who were clients at a health maintenance organization served as comparison group subjects. Forester used hematocrit readings as the measure of treatment effectiveness. During the sixth month of the pregnancy, and again at the 36th-week visit, a hematocrit laboratory test was performed. Data were analyzed by comparing the degree of change that had occurred in the two hematocrit readings within the two groups. The researcher found no significant differences in physiologic anemia in the two groups, as measured by the changes in hematocrit tests.

Review and critique this study. Suggest alternative ways of collecting the data for the research problem. To assist you in your critique, here are some guiding questions:

a. The data in this study were collected by a biophysiologic measure. Could the data have been collected in another way? In your opinion, should they have been?

b. Is the measure used an in vivo or in vitro type of measurement? Is it an invasive or noninvasive type of procedure?

c. Comment on the objectivity of the data collection method. How does its objectivity compare with other methods of measuring the dependent variable (e.g., observations of pallor of the skin, mucous membranes, and fingernail beds)?

d. What other biophysiologic measures might have been used to collect data in the study?

4. Below are several suggested research articles in which a biophysiologic method was used. Review one of the articles, and respond to questions a through d from Question D.3, to the extent possible, in terms of this actual study.

- Chang, Y. J., Anderson, G. C., Dowling, D., & Lin, C. H. (2002). Decreased activity and oxygen desaturation in prone ventilated preterm infants during the first postnatal week. *Heart & Lung, 31,* 34–42.
- Faulkner, M. S., Hathaway, D., & Tolley, B. (2003). Cardiovascular autonomic function in healthy adolescents. *Heart & Lung, 32,* 10–22
- George, E. L., Hofa L. A., Boujoukos, A., & Zullo, T. G. (2002). Effect of positioning on oxygenation in single-lung transplant recipients. *American Journal of Critical Care, 11,* 66–75.
- McCarthy-Becket, D. O. (2002). Dietary supplementation with conjugated linoleic acid does not improve nutritional status of tumor-bearing rats. *Research in Nursing & Health, 25,* 49–57.
- Oliveira, S. M., Arcuri, E. A., & Santos, J. L. (2002). Cuff width influence on blood pressure measurement during the pregnant-puerperal cycle. *Journal of Advanced Nursing, 38,* 180–189.

E. Special Projects

1. Develop a hypothesis in which each of the following could be used as measurements of the dependent variable:

    a. ECG readings
    b. Glucose concentration in the blood
    c. Vital capacity
    d. Body temperature
    e. ACTH levels
    f. Microbiologic culture of sputum
    g. Blood volume

    h. Blood pressure
    i. Red blood cell count
    j. Reaction time

2. Suppose that you wanted to evaluate the effect of an experimental nursing intervention on the well-being and comfort of cardiac patients. Indicate several biophysiologic measures you might consider using in such a study. Evaluate each of your suggestions with respect to ease of obtaining the data, relevance, and objectivity.

3. Suppose that you were studying patients' opinions about the elements of care that are important to them during hospitalization. Develop 25 statements that might be used in a Q sort for such a study. One example might be "Receive explanation about what is being done to me and why."

4. Using procedures described in Chapter 17, suggest ways of collecting data on the following: fear of death among the elderly; body image among amputees; reactions to the onset of menarche; anxiety; quality of life; nurses' morale in an emergency room; and dependence among cerebral palsied children.

CHAPTER **18**

Assessing Data Quality

A. Matching Exercises

1. Match each statement from Set B with one of the phrases from Set A. Indicate the letter corresponding to your response next to each of the statements in Set B.

SET A
a. Reliability
b. Validity
c. Both reliability and validity
d. Neither reliability nor validity

SET B	**RESPONSE**
1. Is concerned with the accuracy of measures	_____
2. The measures must be high on this for the results of a study to be valid	_____
3. If a measure possesses this, then it is necessarily valid	_____
4. Can in some cases be estimated by procedures that yield a quantified coefficient	_____
5. Can be enhanced by lengthening (adding subparts to) the measure	_____
6. Is always improved when the measure is made more efficient	_____
7. May in some cases be assessed by scrutinizing the components (subparts) of the measure	_____
8. Is necessarily high when the measure is high on objectivity	_____
9. Represents the proportion of true variability in a measure to total obtained variability	_____

10. Is concerned with whether the researcher has adequately conceptualized the variables under investigation   _____

2. Match each statement from Set B with one of the phrases from Set A. Indicate the letter corresponding to your response next to each of the statements in Set B.

SET A
a. Data triangulation
b. Investigator triangulation
c. Theory triangulation
d. Method triangulation

SET B   **RESPONSE**

1. A researcher studying health beliefs of the rural elderly interviews old people and health care providers in the area.   _____

2. A researcher tests narrative data, collected in interviews with people who attempted suicide, against two alternative explanations of stress and coping.   _____

3. Two researchers independently interview 10 informants in a study of adjustment to a cancer diagnosis, and debrief with each other to review what they have learned.   _____

4. A researcher studying school-based clinics observes interactions in the clinics and also conducts in-depth interviews with students.   _____

5. A researcher studying the process of resolving an infertility problem interviews husbands and wives separately.   _____

6. Themes emerging in the field notes of an observer on a psychiatric ward are categorized and labeled independently by the researcher and an assistant.   _____

B. Completion Exercises

Write the words or phrases that correctly complete the following sentences.

1. People are not measured directly; their _____ are measured.

2. The procedure known as _____ refers to the assignment of numerical information to indicate how much of an attribute is present.

3. In measurement, numbers are assigned according to specified

   _____ .

4. Obtained scores almost always consist of an error component and a(n)

   _____ component.

5. From a measurement perspective, response-set biases represent a source of

   _____ .

6. A reliable measure is one that maximizes the _____ component of observed scores.

7. Test-retest reliability focuses on the _____ of a measure.

8. A(n) _____ is an index of the strength and direction of a relationship between two variables.

9. The relationship between number of years of nursing experience and hourly wage would be expected to be a _____ relationship.

10. A correlation of 1.00 indicates a _____ relationship between two variables.

11. When the values on one variable tend to be high among individuals who score low on a second variable, the relationship is described as _____.

12. Another term for internal consistency is _____ .

13. Procedures that examine the proportion of agreements between two independent judges yield estimates of _____ .

14. An instrument that is not reliable cannot be _____ .

15. A measure that looks as though it is measuring what it purports to measure is said to have _____ validity.

16. The type of validity that focuses on the representativeness of the measure's individual items is _____ validity.

17. The type of validity that deals with the ability of an instrument to distinguish individuals who differ in terms of some future criterion is _____ validity.

18. _____ refers to evidence that different methods of measuring a concept yield comparable results.

19. _____ refers to evidence that a concept being measured is different from other similar concepts.

20. _____ is the ability of a screening instrument to identify cases correctly and _____ is its ability to identify noncases correctly.

21. An instrument that makes good use of the time required to obtain measurements is described as _____ .

22. An instrument that can make fine discriminations for different amounts of an attribute is described as high on _____ .

23. The four criteria for establishing the trustworthiness of qualitative data are _____, _____, _____, and _____ .

24. When qualitative researchers undertake _____ in the field, they have more opportunity to develop trust with informants and to explore possible misinformation.

25. The use of multiple sources of information in a study as a means of verification is known as _____ .

26. _____ is the technique of debriefing with informants to evaluate the credibility of the analysis of qualitative data.

27. The criterion of _____ refers to the objectivity or neutrality of the data.

28. In qualitative studies, a(n)_____ of data and documents by an independent reviewer can verify the dependability and neutrality of the data and their interpretation.

C. Study Questions

1. Define the following terms. Compare your definition with the definition in Chapter 18 or in the glossary of the textbook.

    a. Measurement: _____

    _____

b. Isomorphism: _____

_____

c. Obtained score: _____

_____

d. Error of measurement: _____

_____

e. Reliability: _____

_____

f. Test-retest reliability: _____

_____

g. Reliability coefficient: _____

_____

h. Internal consistency: _____

_____

i. Spearman-Brown prophecy formula: _____

_____

j. Cronbach's alpha: _____

_____

k. Interrater reliability: _____

_____

l. Validity: _____

_____

m. Content validity: _____

_____

n. Criterion-related validity: _____

_____

o. Construct validity: _____

_____

p. Known-groups technique: _____

_____

q. Multitrait-multimethod matrix: _____

_____

r. Triangulation: _____

_____

s. Audit trail: _____

_____

t. Credibility: _____

_____

u. Persistent observation: _____

_____

v. Transferability:_____

_____

w. Psychometric assessment: _____

_____

2. Use the Spearman-Brown prophecy formula to compute the following:

   a. The full reliability of a 12-item scale whose split-half reliability (i.e., based on six items) is .62. _____

   b. The approximate number of items that would have to be added to increase the reliability of a scale from .70 (for 10 items) to .85. _____

   c. The decrease in reliability for a scale with 30 items and a reliability of .90 if five items were eliminated. _____

3. The reliability of measures of which of the following attributes would *not* be appropriately assessed using a test-retest procedure with 1 month between administrations? Why?

   a. Attitudes toward abortion: _____

   _____

   b. Stress: _____

   _____

   c. Achievement motivation: _____

   _____

    d. Nursing effectiveness: _____

_____

    e. Depression: _____

_____

4. Comment on the meaning and implications of the following statement:

    A researcher found that the internal consistency of her 20-item scale measuring attitudes toward nurse-midwives was .74, using the Cronbach alpha formula.

5. In the following situation, what might be some of the sources of measurement error?

    One hundred nurses who worked in a large metropolitan hospital were asked to complete a 10-item Likert scale designed to measure job satisfaction. The questionnaires were distributed by nursing supervisors at the end of shifts. The staff nurses were asked to complete the forms and return them immediately to their supervisors.

6. Identify what is incorrect about the following statements:

    a. "My scale is highly reliable, so it must be valid."

_____

_____

    b. "My instrument yielded an internal consistency coefficient of .80, so it must be stable."

_____

_____

    c. "The validity coefficient between my scale and a criterion measure was .40; therefore, my scale must be of low validity."

_____

_____

    d. "My scale had a reliability coefficient of .80. Therefore, an obtained score of 20 is indicative of a true score of 16."

_____

_____

    e. "The validation study proved that my measure has construct validity."

_____

_____

   f. "My measure of stress was highly reliable in my study of primiparous women; you should use it in your study of stress among emergency room staff."

   _____

   _____

   g. "My advisor examined my new measure of dependence in nursing home residents and, based on its content, assured me the measure was valid."

   _____

   _____

7. What aspects of the multitrait-multimethod matrix that follows identify weaknesses in the measures?

	Traits	Method 1		Method 2	
		A_1	B_1	A_2	B_2
Method 1	A_1	(.40)			
	B_1	.38	(.65)		
Method 2	A_2	.36	.50	(.80)	
	B_2	.19	.48	.25	(.75)

8. Suppose you were going to conduct an ethnographic study to learn about the culture of a pediatric intensive care unit. What measures could you take to enhance the credibility of your study?

9. Suppose you were conducting a grounded theory study of couples' coming to terms with infertility. What might you do to incorporate various types of triangulation into your study?

D. Application Exercises

1. A brief summary of a fictitious study is presented next. Read the summary and then respond to the questions that follow.

   Milot (2003) wanted to study paternal bonding and attachment among men who had recently become fathers. Her main objective was to compare paternal attachment among men who had participated with their wives in prenatal classes and were present during childbirth with men who had not. In reviewing prior work in this area, Milot was unable to identify a paternal attachment scale that she found suitable to her needs. Therefore, she developed her own scale to measure paternal attachment. Her scale consisted of 10 statements that respondents were asked to rate as "very much like me," "somewhat like me," or "not at all like me." An example of the statements on the scale is, "The birth of my baby aroused sentiments of immediate affection and pride." Total scores were obtained by using procedures for summated rating scales. Milot pretested her scale with 30 men within 48 hours of the delivery of their babies. The internal consistency of the scale was assessed using the split-half technique, which, when corrected using the Spearman-Brown formula, yielded a reliability coefficient of .62. In terms of validating the instrument, Milot used two approaches. First, she invited two colleagues who worked in maternal-child nursing to review the 10 statements and evaluate them in terms of content validity. Second, she asked nurses who worked in the hospital maternity ward to provide ratings, on a 0 to 10 scale, of how attached each new father appeared to be, based on the nurses' observations of the fathers' behavior regarding their babies. The correlations between the fathers' scale scores and the nurses' ratings was .56.

Review and critique this research effort. Suggest alternative ways of assessing the reliability and validity of the instrument. To assist you in your critique, here are some guiding questions:

a. What method was used to assess the reliability of the instrument? On what aspect of reliability does this method focus? Is this focus appropriate? Should some alternative method for estimating reliability have been used? Should an *additional* method of estimating reliability have been used?

b. Comment on the adequacy of the instrument's reliability. Should the reliability be better? If so, what might the researcher do to improve the reliability?

c. What method was used to assess the validity of the instrument? On what aspect of validity does this approach focus? Is this focus appropriate? Should some alternative method for estimating validity have been used? Should an *additional* method of estimating validity have been used?

d. Comment on the adequacy of the instrument's validity. Should the validity be better? If so, what might the researcher do to improve the validity?

e. Comment on the efficiency, precision, objectivity, and reactivity of the instrument.

2. Below are several suggested research articles. Read one of these articles, paying special attention to the ways the researchers assessed the adequacy of their measuring tool. Evaluate the measurement strategy, using questions a through e from Question D.1 as a guide. (Ignore the more technical aspects of the report, such as those that deal with factor analysis.)

- Barrosso, J., Lynn, M. R. (2002). Psychometric properties of the HIV-Related Fatigue Scale. *Journal of the Association of Nurses in AIDS Care, 13,* 66–75.
- Byrne, M. W., & Keefe, M. R. (2003). Comparison of two measures of parent-child interaction. *Nursing Research, 52,* 34–41.
- Reece, S. M., & Harkless, G. E. (2002). Testing of the PHS-ES: A measure of Perimenopausal Health Self-Efficacy. *Journal of Nursing Measurement, 10,* 15–26.
- Ryden, M. B., Gross, C. R., Savik, K., Snyder, M., Oh, H. L., Jang, Y., Wang, J., Krichbaum, K. E. (2000). Development of a measure of resident satisfaction with the nursing home. *Research in Nursing & Health, 23,* 237–245.

- Wells, D. K., James, K., Stewart, J. L., Moore, I. M., Kelly, K. P., Moore, B., Bond, D., Diamond, J., Hall, B., Mahan, R., Roll, L., & Speckhart, B. (2002). The care of my child with cancer: A new instrument to measure caregiving demand in parents of children with cancer. *Journal of Pediatric Nursing, 17,* 201–210.

3. Below is a brief description of a fictitious study, followed by a critique. Do you agree with the critique? Can you add other comments relevant to issues discussed in Chapter 18 of the textbook?

Fictitious Study. Guslander (2003) developed a 12-item Likert scale that measured feelings of loneliness and social isolation among the elderly. Examples of the items include, "I have lots of friends with whom I am close" and "Sometimes days go by without my having a real conversation with anyone." Guslander pretested her instrument with 50 men and women aged 65 to 75 years living independently in the community. She estimated the reliability of the scale using internal consistency procedures (Cronbach's alpha), which yielded a reliability coefficient of .61.

Guslander took two steps to validate her scale. First, she asked two geriatric nurses to examine the 12 items to assess the scale's content validity. These experts suggested some wording changes on three items and recommended replacing one other. Next, she compared the scale scores of 100 elderly widows and widowers with 100 elderly married men and women. Her rationale was that the widowed would probably feel lonelier as a group than the nonwidowed. Her expectation was confirmed. Guslander concluded that her scale was reasonably valid and reliable.

Critique. Guslander took some reasonable steps in constructing her scale and assessing its quality. For example, it appears that she included a sufficient number of items (12) to yield discriminating scores. She used the Cronbach's alpha approach, which is the best method available for assessing the internal consistency of Likert scales.

The reliability of Guslander's scale, however, could and should be improved. The reliability coefficient of .61 suggests that there is considerable measurement error. There are several steps that Guslander could take to try to raise the reliability. First, she could make sure that each item on her scale is doing the job it was intended to do. Remember that scales are designed to discriminate among people who possess different amounts of some trait, in this case social isolation. If Guslander identifies one or more items for which there is little variability (i.e., most respondents either agree or disagree), then the item should be discarded. It is probably not measuring social isolation if everyone responds the same way. Guslander should also consider lengthening the scale. Other things being equal, longer scales are more reliable than shorter ones.

Guslander's efforts to validate her scale also deserve comment. Her first step was to consider the content validity of the scale. Having two knowledgeable people examine the scale was a desirable thing to do. Nevertheless, it cannot be said that this activity in itself ensured the validity of the scale. As a second step, Guslander used the known-groups technique. The data she obtained provided some useful evidence of the scale's construct validity. After making some of the revisions suggested above to improve the scale's reliability, however, Guslander would do well to gather some additional data to support the scale's construct validity. For example, one might suspect that people would feel less socially isolated if they reported having kin living within a 20-mile radius; if they had visited with a friend within a 72-hour period preceding the completion of the scale; and if they were active members of a club, church group, or other social organization. All of these expectations could be tested. If Guslander took these additional steps to establish the reliability and validity of her scale and obtained favorable results, she could be more confident that the quality of her scale was high.

4. Below are several suggested research reports on qualitative studies. Read and critique one of these articles, paying special attention to the ways in which the researcher addressed data quality issues. To assist you in your critique, here are some guiding questions:

   a. Does the report discuss efforts the researcher made to enhance and appraise data quality? Is the documentation regarding efforts to assess data quality sufficiently detailed and clear?
   b. What were those efforts? Was any type of triangulation used? Were there member checks? Was there an external audit of the data?
   c. How adequate were the procedures that were used? What other techniques could have been used profitably to enhance and assess data quality? How much confidence do the researcher's efforts inspire regarding data quality?
   d. Given the procedures that were used to enhance data quality, what can you conclude about the credibility, transferability, dependability, and confirmability of the data?

   - Erwin, E. (2002). Adolescent perceptions of relevant social problems. *Journal of Child & Adolescent Psychiatric Nursing, 15,* 24–34.
   - Neufeld, A., Harrison, M. J., Stewart, M. J., Hughes, K. D., & Spitzer, D. (2002). Immigrant women: Making connections to community resources for support in family caregiving. *Qualitative Health Research, 12,* 751–768.
   - Weiss, M. E., Saks, N. P., & Harris, S. (2002). Resolving the uncertainty of preterm symptoms: Women's experiences with the onset of preterm labor. *Journal of Obstetric, Gynecologic, and Neonatal Nursing, 31,* 66–76.
   - Wise, B. V. (2002). In their own words: The lived experience of pediatric liver transplantation. *Qualitative Health Research, 12,* 74–90.
   - Whittemore, R., Chase, S. K., Mandle, C. L., & Roy, Sr. C. (2002). Lifestyle change in type 2 diabetes. *Nursing Research, 51* 18–25.

E. Special Projects

1. Suppose that you were developing an instrument to measure attitudes toward human cloning. Your measure consists of 15 Likert-type items. Describe what you would do to: (a) estimate the reliability of your scale and (b) assess the validity of your scale.

2. Suggest the type of groups that might be used to validate measures of the following concepts using the known-groups technique:

   a. Self-esteem
   b. Empathy
   c. Capacity for self-care
   d. Emotional dependence
   e. Depression
   f. Hopelessness
   g. Health-promoting practices
   h. Health motivation
   i. Body image
   j. Coping capacity

3. Suppose you were interested in conducting an in-depth study of the experiences of women who had been raped. Describe ways in which you would establish the trustworthiness of your data and interpretations of them.

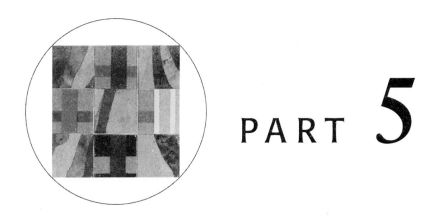

PART 5

The Analysis of
Research Data

CHAPTER **19**

Analyzing Quantitative Data: Descriptive Statistics

A. Matching Exercises

1. Match each variable in Set B with the level of measurement from Set A that captures the highest possible level for that variable. Indicate the letter corresponding to your response next to each variable in Set B.

SET A
a. Nominal scale
b. Ordinal scale
c. Interval scale
d. Ratio scale

SET B   **RESPONSE**

1. Hours spent in labor before childbirth   _____

2. Religious affiliation   _____

3. Reaction time   _____

4. Marital status   _____

5. Temperature on the centigrade scale   _____

6. Nursing specialty area   _____

7. Status on the following scale: nonsmoker; light smoker; heavy smoker   _____

8. Pulse rate   _____

9. Score on a 25-item Likert scale   _____

10. Highest degree or certification attained   _____

11. Apgar scores   _____

12. Membership in the American Nurses' Association   _____

2. Match each statement or phrase from Set B with one of the phrases from Set A. Indicate the letter corresponding to your response next to each of the statements in Set B.

SET A

a. Measure(s) of central tendency
b. Measure(s) of variability
c. Measure(s) of neither central tendency nor variability
d. Measure(s) of both central tendency and variability

SET B	**RESPONSE**
1. The range	_____
2. In lay terms, an average	_____
3. A percentage	_____
4. A parameter	_____
5. Descriptor(s) of a distribution of scores	_____
6. Descriptor(s) of how heterogeneous a set of values is	_____
7. A standard deviation	_____
8. The mode	_____
9. Can be plotted on histograms	_____
10. Coincide in a normal distribution	_____

B. Completion Exercises

Write the words or phrases that correctly complete the following sentences.

1. Nominal measurement involves a simple _____ of objects according to some criterion.

2. Rank-order questions are an example of _____ measures.

3. With ratio-level measures, there is a real, rational _____ .

4. Unlike ordinal measures, interval measures involve _____ between points on the scale.

5. A descriptive index (e.g., percentage) from a sample is called a(n) _____ used to estimate a population _____.

6. Researchers using quantitative analysis apply _____ to draw conclusions about a population based on information from a sample.

7. A(n) _____ is a systematic arrangement of quantitative data from lowest to highest values.

8. In the equation $f = N$, the N represents the total _____ .

9. Histograms and _____ are the two most common ways of presenting frequency information in graphic form.

10. A distribution is described as _____ if the two halves are mirror images of each other.

11. A distribution is _____ skewed if its longer tail points to the left.

12. A distribution that has only one peak is said to be _____ .

13. Many human characteristics such as height and intelligence are distributed to approximate a(n) _____ .

14. Measures that summarize the "typical" value in a distribution are known as measures of _____ .

15. The symbol $\bar{X}$ is usually used by researchers to designate the _____ .

16. In a positively skewed distribution, the index indicating the "average" value that would be the farthest of the three indexes to the left would be the _____ .

17. Measures of _____ are concerned with how spread out data are.

18. When scores are not very spread out (i.e., dispersed over a wide range of values), the sample is said to be _____ with respect to that variable.

19. The _____ indicates one half of the range of scores within which the middle 50% of the scores lie.

20. The difference between an individual raw score and the mean is known as a(n) _____ .

21. A squared standard deviation is referred to as a(n) _____ .

22. Statistics for two variables examined simultaneously are called _____ .

23. Another term for a contingency table is a(n) _____ .

24. A graphic representation of a correlation between two variables is referred to as a(n) _____ .

25. The most commonly used correlation index is _____ .

C. Study Questions

1. Define the following terms. Compare your definition with the definition in Chapter 19 or in the glossary of the textbook.

   a. Nominal measurement: _____

   _____

   b. Ordinal measurement: _____

   _____

   c. Interval-level measurement: _____

   _____

   d. Ratio measurement: _____

   _____

   e. Parameter: _____

   _____

   f. Histogram: _____

   _____

   g. Skewed distribution: _____

   _____

   h. Bimodal distribution: _____

   _____

   i. Normal distribution: _____

   _____

   j. Mode: _____

   _____

   k. Median: _____

   _____

   l. Mean: _____

   _____

   m. Range: _____

   _____

   n. Standard deviation: _____

   _____

o. Contingency table: _____

_____

p. Correlation matrix: _____

_____

2. For each of the following variables, specify the *highest* possible level of measurement that a researcher could attain.

a. Attitudes toward the mentally handicapped _____

b. Birth order _____

c. Length of labor _____

d. White blood cell count _____

e. Blood type _____

f. Tidal volume _____

g. Scholastic Aptitude Test (SAT) scores _____

h. Unit assignment for nursing staff _____

i. Motivation for achievement _____

j. Amount of sputum _____

3. Prepare a frequency distribution and histogram for the following set of data values, which represent the ages of 30 women receiving estrogen replacement therapy:

47 50 51 50 48 51 50 51 49 51
54 49 49 53 51 52 51 52 50 53
49 51 52 51 50 55 48 54 53 52

Describe the resulting distribution in terms of its symmetry and modality.

4. Calculate the mean, median, and mode for the following pulse rates:

78 84 69 98 102 72 87 75 79 84 88 84 83 71 73

Mean: _____ Median: _____ Mode: _____

5. At the top of page 186 is a contingency table from an SPSS printout. The table presents data from a study of sexually active teenagers in which both males and females were asked how old they were when they first had sexual intercourse. Each row in the table indicates the ages specified by the respondents. The last row contains the code for respondents who could not remember how old they were. Answer the following questions about this contingency table:

			GENDER		
			Male	Female	Total
AGE	13	Count	1	2	3
		% within AGE	33.3%	66.7%	100.0%
		% within GENDER	2.2%	4.4%	3.3%
		% of Total	1.1%	2.2%	3.3%
	14	Count	6	3	9
		% within AGE	66.7%	33.3%	100.0%
		% within GENDER	13.3%	6.7%	10.0%
		% of Total	6.7%	3.3%	10.0%
	15	Count	9	6	15
		% within AGE	60.0%	40.0%	100.0%
		% within GENDER	20.0%	13.3%	16.7%
		% of Total	10.0%	6.7%	16.7%
	16	Count	15	10	25
		% within AGE	60.0%	40.0%	100.0%
		% within GENDER	33.3%	22.2%	27.8%
		% of Total	16.7%	11.1%	27.8%
	17	Count	11	14	25
		% within AGE	44.0%	56.0%	100.0%
		% within GENDER	24.4%	31.1%	27.8%
		% of Total	12.2%	15.6%	27.8%
	18	Count	2	8	10
		% within AGE	20.0%	80.0%	100.0%
		% within GENDER	4.4%	17.8%	11.1%
		% of Total	2.2%	8.9%	11.1%
	Don't Remember	Count	1	2	3
		% within AGE	33.3%	66.7%	100.0%
		% within GENDER	2.2%	4.4%	3.3%
		% of Total	1.1%	2.2%	3.3%
Total		Count	45	45	90
		% within AGE	50.0%	50.0%	100.0%
		% within GENDER	100.0%	100.0%	100.0%
		% of Total	50.0%	50.0%	100.0%

a. How many males were included in the study? _____

b. How many females first had sexual intercourse at age 14? _____

c. What percentage of respondents were 16 years of age when they first had sexual intercourse? _____

   d. What percentage of males did not know at what age they first had sexual intercourse? _____

   e. Of those respondents who were 13 years of age when they first had sexual intercourse, what percentage was female? _____

6. Write out the meaning of each of the following symbols:

   a. Σ _____

   b. $\bar{X}$ _____

   c. f _____

   d. N _____

   e. X _____

   f. x _____

   g. SD _____

7. Suppose a researcher has conducted a study concerning lactose intolerance in children. The data reveal that 12 boys and 16 girls have lactose intolerance, out of a sample of 60 children of each gender. Construct a contingency table and calculate the row, column, and total percentages for each cell in the table. Discuss the meaning of these statistics.

8. A researcher has collected data on pulse rate and scores on a final examination for 10 students and would like to know if there is a relationship between the two measures. Compute Pearson's r for these data:

        Pulse rate: 84 72 82 68 96 64 92 88 76 74
        Test scores: 92 84 88 72 68 74 72 90 82 86

D. Application Exercises

1. Here is a brief summary of a fictitious study. Read the summary and then respond to the questions that follow.

   Joyce (2003) hypothesized that sleeping problems in infants were related to various conditions and experiences during childbirth. Fifty infants aged 3 to 6 months were diagnosed as having severe sleep disturbance problems. A group of 50 infants aged 3 to 6 months who had normal sleeping patterns was used as the comparison group. Joyce obtained the hospital records for all 100 children. The two groups were compared in terms of the following variables: amount of anesthesia administered during labor and delivery (none, small amount, large amount); length of time in labor (number of hours and minutes); type of delivery (cesarean or vaginal); birth weight (in grams); and Apgar scores at 3 minutes (score from 1 to 10). Joyce found that the sleep disturbance group had longer time in labor than the comparison group. The groups were comparable in terms of the other variables.

Review and critique this research effort. Suggest alternative measurement approaches. To assist you in your critique, here are some guiding questions:

    a. How many variables were measured in this study?

    b. For each variable, identify the level of measurement that was used.

    c. For each variable, indicate whether the measurement could have been made at a higher level of measurement than the level that was used. If yes, specify how you might measure the variable to obtain a higher level measure.

    d. For two of the variables, write out operational definitions that clearly indicate the rules of measurement for those variables.

2. Below are several suggested research articles. Skim one or more of these articles, paying special attention to the ways in which the research variables were operationalized. Evaluate the researcher's measurement strategy, using questions a through d from Question D.1 as a guide.

   - Bieniasz, M. E., Underwood, D., Bailey, J., & Ruffin, M. T. (2003). Women's feedback on a chemopreventive trial for cervical dysplasia. *Applied Nursing Research,* 16, 22–28.
   - Carruth, A. K., Skarke, L., Moffett, B., & Prestholdt, C. (2002). Nonfatal injury experiences among women on family farms. *Clinical Nursing Research, 11,* 130–148.
   - Johnson, T. S. (2003). Hypoglycemia and the full-term newborn: How well does birth weight for gestational age predict risk? *Journal of Obstetric, Gynecologic, and Neonatal Nursing, 32,* 48–57.
   - Stark, M. A. (2000). Is it difficult to concentrate during the 3rd trimester and postpartum? *Journal of Obstetric, Gynecologic, and Neonatal Nursing, 29,* 378–389.
   - Walker, L. O., & Kim, M. (2002). Psychosocial thriving during late pregnancy: Relationship to ethnicity, gestational weight gain, and birth weight. *Journal of Obstetric, Gynecologic, and Neonatal Nursing, 31,* 263–274.
   - Wilson, D. (2002). The duration and degree of end-of-life dependency of home care clients and hospital inpatients. *Applied Nursing Research, 15,* 81–86.

3. Here is a brief summary of the descriptive analyses of another fictitious study. Read the summary and then respond to the questions that follow.

   Portnoy (2002) hypothesized that patients with a high degree of physical mobility would perceive themselves as being healthier than patients with less physical mobility. To test this hypothesis, 120 male patients in a Veterans' Administration hospital were asked to rate themselves on a five-point scale regarding their current physical health (1 = very unhealthy and 5 = very healthy) and to predict the number of days that they would be hospitalized. Forty of these patients had been categorized as "limited mobility," another 40 were classified as "moderate mobility," and the remaining 40 were described as "high mobility." Portnoy reported a portion of her findings as follows:

The self-ratings of physical health were fairly normally distributed for the sample as a whole: 42% rated themselves as neither healthy nor unhealthy; 7% and 21% described themselves as "very healthy" or "somewhat healthy," respectively. At the other extreme, 6% said they were "very unhealthy," and 24% said "somewhat unhealthy." The three groups differed in their ratings, however. In the high-mobility group, 45% said they were either "very" or "somewhat" healthy, while only 30% of the moderate-mobility and 15% of the low-mobility groups said this. For the entire sample, the mean predicted length of stay was 14.1 days. The median length, however, was only 12.5 days. For the three groups, the means and standard deviations with respect to predicted length of stay in hospital were as follows:

Group	Mean	Standard Deviation
High Mobility	7.1	3.2
Moderate Mobility	11.9	4.5
Low Mobility	23.3	7.4

In this sample of patients, the correlation between predicted length of stay in hospital and the health rating was .56.

Review and critique this study, particularly with respect to the statistical analysis. To assist you in this critique, here are some guiding questions:

a. Was the mode of data analysis (i.e., quantitative versus qualitative) appropriate? Why or why not?

b. Which of the following types of statistical analysis were used in this example?

Frequency distribution
Measure of central tendency
Measure of variability
Contingency table
Correlation

c. Comment on the appropriateness of each statistic reported in the example. Is the statistic appropriate given the level of measurement of the variable? Does the statistic throw away information? Is the statistic the most stable statistic possible?

d. Identify two or three statistics that were not reported by the researcher that could have been reported given the data that were collected. Evaluate the extent to which the absence of this information weakened (or streamlined) the report of the results.

e. Discuss the meaning of the means and standard deviations reported in this example.

4. Below are several suggested research articles. Skim one (or more) of these articles, and respond to questions a through e from Question D.3 in terms of the

actual research study. (At this point, ignore the references to tests of statistical significance, which are covered in the next chapter.)

- Low, G., & Gutman, G. (2003). Couples' ratings of chronic obstructive pulmonary disease patients' quality of life. *Clinical Nursing Research, 12,* 28–48.
- Mayo, A. M., Chang, B. L., & Omery, A. (2002). Use of protocols and guidelines by telephone nurses. *Clinical Nursing Research, 11,* 204–219.
- Morin, K. H., Brogan, S., & Flavin, S. K. (2002). Attitudes and perceptions of body image in postpartum African American women. *MCN: The Journal of Maternal/Child Nursing, 27,* 20–25.
- Plach, S. K., & Heidrich, S. M. (2002). Social role quality, physical health, and psychological well-being in women after heart surgery. *Research in Nursing & Health, 25,* 189–202.

SUBJECT NO.	SHIFT[a]	ANXIETY SCORES[b]	SUPERVISOR'S PERFORMANCE RATING[c]	NO. OF YEARS OF EXPERIENCE	MARITAL STATUS[d]	JOB SATISFACTION SCORE[e]
1	1	10	4	5	2	4
2	1	13	4	2	2	5
3	1	8	2	1	1	3
4	1	4	7	10	1	3
5	1	6	9	12	1	4
6	1	9	8	7	1	2
7	1	12	6	8	2	4
8	1	5	4	2	1	5
9	2	10	5	4	2	1
10	2	14	6	1	2	4
11	2	8	5	3	1	5
12	2	15	8	2	2	2
13	2	11	8	7	2	3
14	2	14	7	9	1	1
15	2	1	5	3	2	2
16	2	8	8	6	1	3
17	3	3	7	19	2	4
18	3	7	4	7	1	1
19	3	19	5	1	2	2
20	3	5	6	11	1	1
21	3	8	3	2	1	3
22	3	10	4	5	2	2
23	3	13	6	6	2	1
24	3	14	5	3	1	2

[a]1 = day; 2 = evening; 3 = night
[b]Scores are from a low of 0 to a high of 20, 20 = most anxious
[c]Ratings are from 1 = poor to 9 = excellent
[d]1 = married; 2 = not married
[e]Scores are from low of 1 to high of 5; 5 = most satisfied

- VanDongen, C. J. (2002). Environmental health and nursing practice: A survey of registered nurses. *Applied Nursing Research, 15*, 67–73.

E. Special Projects

1. Fictitious data from 24 nurses for six variables are presented on the facing page. Compute and present 5 to 10 different statistics that you think would best summarize this information.

2. Ask 25 friends, classmates, or colleagues the following four questions:
   - How many brothers and sisters do you have?
   - How many children do you expect to have in total?
   - Would you describe your family during your childhood as "close" or "not very close"?
   - On your fourteenth birthday, were you living with both biologic parents, primarily with one biologic parent, or with neither biologic parent?

   When you have gathered your data, calculate and present several statistics that describe the information you obtained.

3. Develop a problem statement (or a hypothesis) for a nursing research study. Prepare operational definitions that specify measurement rules for the variables in your statement. Identify for each variable the level of measurement your definition implies.

CHAPTER **20**

Analyzing Quantitative Data: Inferential Statistics

A. *Matching Exercises*

Match each phrase or statement from Set B with one of the phrases in Set A. Indicate the letter corresponding to your response next to each of the statements in Set B.

SET A
a. Parametric test(s)
b. Nonparametric test(s)
c. Neither parametric nor nonparametric tests
d. Both parametric and nonparametric tests

SET B   **RESPONSE**

1. The signed rank test   _____
2. Paired *t*-test   _____
3. Researcher establishes the risk of Type I errors   _____
4. Used when a score distribution is non-normal   _____
5. Offers proof that the null hypothesis is either true or false   _____
6. Assumes the dependent variable is measured on an interval or ratio scale   _____
7. Uses sample data to estimate population values   _____
8. Kruskal-Wallis test   _____
9. Computed statistics are compared to tabled values based on theoretical distributions   _____
10. Used most frequently by nurse researchers   _____
11. Used to compare differences for three groups   _____

12. ANOVA   _____

13. Pearson's *r*   _____

14. Chi-square test   _____

B. Completion Exercises

Write the words or phrases that correctly complete the following sentences.

1. Sampling distributions of means have a _____distribution.

2. The standard error of the mean is estimated by dividing the sample standard deviation by the square root of the _____ .

3. The Greek letter mu (μ) usually symbolizes the _____ .

4. The degree of risk of making a _____ error is controlled by the researcher.

5. Tests that involve the estimation of parameters are referred to as _____tests.

6. The term *distribution-free statistics* is sometimes used for _____ _____tests.

7. The most commonly used _____ are the .05 and .01 levels.

8. Using a .01 rather than a .05 level increases the risk of committing a _____ error.

9. The _____ test is used to compare two groups on the basis of deviations from the median.

10. The statistic computed in an analysis of variance is the _____ statistic.

11. In an analysis of variance, the term analogous to the *variance* is referred to as the _____ .

12. Multifactor ANOVA permits a test of differential effects of one variable for all levels of a second variable, or a test of the_____ hypothesis.

13. The nonparametric test analogous to ANOVA is called the _____ test.

14. In chi-square analyses, observed frequencies are compared with _____ .

15. When both the independent and dependent variables are nominal measures, the most commonly used test statistic is the _____ .

16. Kendall's tau is used when both the independent and dependent variables are _____ measures.

17. A(n) _____ test would be used to compare the heart rates of two groups at three points in time.

18. The _____ is an index describing the magnitude of relationship between two dichotomous variables.

19. If a research report stated that a statistical test yielded a $p > .05$, the result would generally be considered _____ .

20. In power analysis, the four major factors needed to arrive at a solution are the significance criterion, the power criterion, the sample size, and the _____.

C. Study Questions

1. Define the following terms. Compare your definition with the definition in Chapter 20 or in the glossary of the textbook.

   a. Sampling error: _____

   _____

   b. Sampling distribution: _____

   _____

   c. Standard error of the mean: _____

   _____

   d. Point estimation: _____

   _____

   e. Confidence interval: _____

   _____

   f. Null hypothesis: _____

   _____

   g. Type I error: _____

   _____

h. Type II error: _____

_____

i. Level of significance: _____

_____

j. Statistical significance: _____

_____

k. Nonparametric tests: _____

_____

l. Degrees of freedom: _____

_____

m. *t*-test: _____

_____

n. Analysis of variance: _____

_____

o. Multiple comparison procedures: _____

_____

p. Repeated measures ANOVA: _____

_____

q. Chi-square test: _____

_____

r. Power analysis: _____

_____

2. A nurse researcher measured the amount of time (in minutes) spent in recreational activities by a sample of 200 hospitalized paraplegic patients. She compared male and female patients, as well as those 50 years of age and younger versus those over 50 years of age. The four group means were as follows:

Age	Male	Female
≤ 50	98.2 ($n = 50$)	70.1 ($n = 50$)
> 50	50.8 ($n = 50$)	68.3 ($n = 50$)

A two-way ANOVA yielded the following results:

	F	df
Gender	3.61	1,196
Age group	5.87	1,196
Gender × Age group	6.96	1,196

Determine the levels of significance of these results, and interpret their meaning.

3. The correlation between the number of days absent per year and annual salary in a sample of 100 employees of an insurance company was found to be −.23. Discuss this result in terms of significance levels and meaning.

4. Indicate which statistical test(s) you would use to analyze data for the following variables:

a. Variable 1 is psychiatric patients' gender; variable 2 is whether or not the patient has attempted suicide in the past 12 months.

_____

_____

b. Variable 1 is the participation versus nonparticipation of patients with a pulmonary embolus in a special treatment group; variable 2 is the pH of the patients' arterial blood gases.

_____

_____

c. Variable 1 is serum creatinine concentration levels; variable 2 is daily urine output.

_____

_____

d. Variable 1 is patients' marital status (married versus not married); variable 2 is the patients' degrees of self-reported depression (mild versus moderate versus severe).

_____

_____

5. On the next page is a correlation matrix produced by an SPSS run, based on real data from a study of low-income mothers. The variables in this matrix are as follows:

Correlations

Correlations

		R: STRESSFULL LIFE EVENT SCORE	Total Household Income	CES-D Score (Range 0 to 60)	SF12: Physical Health Component Score	SF12: Mental Health Component Score
R: STRESSFUL LIFE EVENT SCORE	Pearson Correlation	1.000	-.024	.275**	-.136**	-.265**
	Sig. (2-tailed)	.	.485	.000	.000	.000
	N	958	887	950	907	907
Total Household Income	Pearson Correlation	-.024	1.000	-.105**	.113**	.055
	Sig. (2-tailed)	.485	.	.002	.001	.113
	N	887	935	893	843	843
CES-D Score (Range 0 to 60)	Pearson Correlation	.275**	-.105**	1.000	-.181**	-.643**
	Sig. (2-tailed)	.000	.002	.	.000	.000
	N	950	893	963	903	903
SF12: Physical Health Component Score	Pearson Correlation	-.136**	.113	-.181**	1.000	.078*
	Sig. (2-tailed)	.000	.001	.000	.	.019
	N	907	843	903	909	909
SF12: Mental Health Component Score	Pearson Correlation	-.265**	.055	-.643**	.078*	1.000
	Sig. (2-tailed)	.000	.113	.000	.019	.
	N	907	843	903	909	909

** Correlation is significiant at the 0.01 level (2-tailed).
* Correlation is significant at the 0.05 level (2-tailed).

- Scores on a scale measuring stressful life events
- Total household income in the prior month
- Scores on the CES-D depression scale
- Scores on the physical health subscale of the SF-12
- Scores on the mental health subscale of the SF-12

Answer the following questions with respect to this matrix:

a. How many respondents completed the stressful life event scale?
b. What is the correlation between total household income and scores on the physical health subscale?
c. Is the correlation between physical health and mental health subscale scores significant at conventional levels?
d. What is the probability that the correlation between depression scores and total household income in this sample is simply a function of chance?
e. With which variable(s) is stressful life event scale scores significantly related at conventional levels?
f. Explain what is meant by the correlation between the depression and mental health scale scores.

D. Application Exercises

1. Below is a brief summary of a fictitious study. Read the summary and then respond to the questions that follow:

Pfeil (2003) investigated whether taste acuity declines with age, using a cross-sectional design. Eighty subjects were given a taste acuity test in which they were asked to indicate, for 25 substances, whether the taste was salty, sweet, bitter, or sour. The substances were presented in randomized order. Each person had five scores: four scores corresponding to the correct identification of the substances in the four taste categories, and one total score. Twenty subjects from each of the following age groups were tested: 31 to 40; 41 to 50; 51 to 60; and 61 to 70. It was hypothesized that taste acuity would decline with age, both overall and for all four subcategories of taste. The mean test scores for the four groups on all five outcome measures are presented below, together with information on the statistical tests performed.

	Age Group (Years)				*F*	*df*	*p*
	31–40	*41–50*	*51–60*	*61–70*			
Salty test	6.3	5.8	5.7	5.4	3.5	3,76	<.05
Sweet test	5.0	5.0	5.4	5.2	1.2	3,76	>.05
Bitter test	4.0	4.1	3.7	3.3	2.6	3,76	<.05
Sour test	1.9	2.0	2.0	2.1	0.8	3,76	>.05
Overall test	17.2	16.9	16.8	16.0	2.4	3,76	<.05

Pfeil concluded that her hypothesis was only partially supported by the data.

Review and critique the above study. Suggest possible alternatives for handling the analysis of the data. To assist you in your critique, here are some guiding questions:

 a. For each of the variables, indicate the actual level of measurement as used; now indicate the highest possible level of measurement for each. Is there a discrepancy? If so, can you think of a justification for it?

 b. What statistical test was used to analyze the data? Did the researcher use the appropriate statistical test? If not, what statistical test do you think would be more suitable?

 c. The test statistics shown are associated with a specified p level. Using the tables in the Appendix of the textbook, determine whether these p levels are correct.

 d. Which of the results is statistically significant? Describe the meaning of each statistical test.

2. Below are several suggested research articles. Skim one (or more) of these articles and respond to questions a through d from Question D.1 in terms of the actual research study. (Focus on the bivariate tests if the study also used multivariate procedures, which are described in the next chapter.)

- Hughes, L. C., Robinson, L. A., Cooley, M.E., Nuamah, I., Grobe, S. J., & McCorkle, R. (2002). Describing an episode of home nursing care for elderly postsurgical cancer patients. *Nursing Research, 51,* 110–118.
- Maloni, J. A., Kane, J. H., Suen, L., & Wang, K. (2002). Dysphoria among high-risk pregnant hospitalized women on bed rest: A longitudinal study. *Nursing Research, 51,* 92–99.
- Taylor, G., & Jones, A. (2002). Effects of a culturally sensitive breast self-examination intervention. *Outcomes Management for Nursing Practice, 6,* 73–78.
- Wakefield, B., Mentes, J., Diggelmann, L., & Culp, K. (2002). Monitoring hydration status in elderly veterans. *Western Journal of Nursing Research, 24,* 132–142.
- West, M. M. (2002). Early risk indicators of substance abuse among nurses. *Journal of Nursing Scholarship, 34,* 187–193.

E. Special Projects

1. Below is a list of variables. Assume that you have data from 500 nurses on these variables. Develop two or three hypotheses regarding the relationships among these variables, and indicate what statistical tests you would use to test your hypotheses.

Number of years of nursing experience
Type of employment setting (hospital, nursing school, public school system, industry)

Salary

Marital status

Job satisfaction ("dissatisfied," "neither dissatisfied nor satisfied," or "satisfied")

Number of children under 18 years of age

Gender

Type of nursing preparation (diploma, Associate's, Bachelor's)

2. Using the data presented in Question E.1 of Chapter 19, perform at least two inferential statistical tests. Write a one-paragraph description of the results.

CHAPTER **21**

Analyzing Quantitative Data: Multivariate Statistics

A. Matching Exercises

Match each phrase from Set B with one (or more) of the statistical analyses presented in Set A. Indicate the letter(s) corresponding to your response next to each of the statements in Set B.

SET A
a. Multiple regression analysis
b. Discriminant function analysis
c. Factor analysis
d. Canonical correlation
e. Multivariate ANOVA

SET B	RESPONSE
1. Always involves more than one independent variable	_____
2. Is based on least-squares principles	_____
3. Yields an R^2 statistic	_____
4. Used to reduce variables to a smaller number of dimensions	_____
5. Has more than one dependent variable	_____
6. Yields a Wilks' lambda statistic	_____
7. Is a multivariate statistical procedure	_____
8. May use a procedure known as principal components	_____
9. Involves a dependent variable that is categorical (nominal level)	_____
10. Can involve as few as three variables	_____

B. Completion Exercises

Write the words or phrases that correctly complete the following sentences.

1. In the basic linear regression equation ($Y = a + bX$), b is referred to as the _____, and a is the _____ .

2. In a regression context, the error terms are referred to as _____ .

3. The square of _____ indicates the proportion of variance accounted for in the dependent variable by two or more independent variables.

4. The _____ coefficient is never less than the highest bivariate correlation between the independent variables and the dependent variable.

5. Independent variables are always introduced one at a time in _____ multiple regression.

6. Scores that have been adjusted to have a mean of zero and a standard deviation of one are called _____ .

7. Standardized regression coefficients are referred to as _____ .

8. ANCOVA is shorthand for _____ .

9. In ANCOVA, the extraneous variable being controlled is referred to as the _____ .

10. _____ is the procedure that yields mean scores on the dependent variable adjusted for covariates.

11. In factor analysis, the underlying dimensions are referred to as _____ .

12. The first phase in factor analysis is the _____ phase, and the second phase is the _____ phase.

13. In factor analysis, _____ are values equal to the sum of the squared weights for each factor.

14. In _____ rotation, factors are kept at right angles to one another, while in _____ rotation, the factors are allowed to be correlated.

15. The procedure known as _____ can be used for classification purposes.

16. The most general multivariate procedure is _____ .

17. MANOVA is the acronym for _____ .

18. In path analysis, the conceptual causal model is depicted in a _____ .

19. A variable whose determinants lie outside of a model in path analysis is called _____ .

20. When a causal flow is unidirectional, the model is said to be _____ .

21. An alternative estimation procedure to ordinary least squares is the _____ procedure.

22. When the dependent variable is a measure of the duration of some event or characteristic, an analytic procedure that can be used is_____ analysis.

23. The acronym for the technique referred to as linear structural relation analysis is _____ .

24. A _____ variable is an unmeasured variable that corresponds to an abstract construct of interest to the researcher.

C. Study Questions

1. Define the following terms. Compare your definition with the definition in Chapter 21 or in the glossary of the textbook.

   a. Multivariate statistics: _____

   _____

   b. Multiple regression analysis: _____

   _____

   c. Least-squares principle: _____

   _____

   d. Coefficient of determination: _____

   _____

e. Analysis of covariance: _____

_____

f. Factor analysis: _____

_____

g. Factor loadings: _____

_____

h. Factor scores: _____

_____

i. Discriminant analysis: _____

_____

j. Canonical correlation: _____

_____

k. Multivariate analysis of variance: _____

_____

l. Path analysis: _____

_____

m. Mediating variable: _____

_____

n. Eta-squared: _____

_____

o. Life table analysis: _____

_____

p. LISREL: _____

_____

q. Measurement model: _____

_____

r. Logistic regression: _____

_____

s. Odds ratio: _____

_____

2. Examine the correlation matrix below and explain the various entries. Explain why the *multiple* correlation coefficient between variables B through E and Satisfaction With Nursing Care (variable A) is .54. Could it be smaller? How could it be made larger? What is the R^2 for the correlation between Satisfaction With Nursing Care and the other variables? What does this mean?

	A Satisfaction With Nursing Care	B Age	C Depression Scores	D Length of Hospital Stay	E Educational Level
Variable A	1.00				
Variable B	−.26	1.00			
Variable C	−.48	.29	1.00		
Variable D	−.19	.22	.68	1.00	
Variable E	.10	−.07	−.17	−.24	1.00

3. Suggest possible covariates that could be used in analyses to study:

   a. The effect of family stress on the incidence of child abuse:

   _____

   _____

   b. The effect of age on patients' acceptance of pastoral counseling:

   _____

   _____

   c. The effect of therapeutic touch on patients' perceptions of well-being:

   _____

   _____

   d. The effect of need for achievement on students' attrition from a nursing program:

   _____

   _____

4. In the following examples, which multivariate procedure is most appropriate for analyzing the data?

   a. A researcher is testing the effect of verbal expressiveness, self-esteem, age, and the availability of family supports among a group of recently discharged psychiatric patients on recidivism (i.e., whether they will be readmitted within 12 months after discharge).

   _____

   _____

b. A researcher is comparing the bereavement and coping processes (as measured on an interval-level scale) of recently widowed versus recently divorced individuals, controlling for their age and length of marriage.

_____

_____

c. A researcher wants to test the effects of (a) two drug treatments and (b) two dosages of each drug on (a) blood pressure and (b) the pH and P_{O_2} levels of arterial blood gases.

_____

_____

d. A researcher wants to predict hospital staff absentee rates based on month of the year, staff rank, shift, number of years with the hospital, and marital status.

_____

_____

5. Below is a list of variables that a nurse researcher might be interested in predicting. For each, suggest at least three independent variables that could be used in a multiple regression analysis.

a. Amount of time spent exercising weekly among teenagers:

_____

_____

b. Nurses' frequency of administering pain medication:

_____

_____

c. Body mass index (a common measure of obesity):

_____

_____

d. Patients' level of fatigue:

_____

_____

e. Anxiety levels of prostatectomy patients:

_____

_____

6. Wang, Redeker, Moreyra, and Diamond, in their 2001 study (*Clinical Nursing Research, 10,* 29–38), used a series of *t*-tests and chi-squared tests to compare two groups of patients who underwent cardiac catheterization with regard to measures of safety, comfort, and satisfaction: those with 4 hours versus 6 hours of bed rest. Identify two or three multivariate procedures that could have been used to analyze the data, being as specific as possible (e.g., if you suggest ANCOVA, identify appropriate covariates).

D. Application Exercises

1. Here is a brief summary of the analyses used in a fictitious study. Read the summary and then respond to the questions that follow.

Masie (2003) studied psychological distress and life satisfaction in a sample of 100 infertile couples. She hypothesized that the individuals' psychological reactions would differ depending on whether the fertility problem was their own or that of their partners. She further hypothesized that women would be more negatively affected psychologically than men by the fertility problem. Masie administered anonymous questionnaires to both husbands and wives who were patients at an infertility clinic. In 50 couples, the fertility problem was diagnosed as a male problem, and in the remaining 50 couples, it was diagnosed as a female problem. The questionnaire included a set of 45 items, designed to measure psychological well-being. The items included such statements as, "I have felt moments of severe depression lately" and, "My husband (wife) and I have been less communicative than usual." Respondents were asked to indicate whether each statement was "very much like me," "somewhat like me," or "not at all like me." Responses to the 45 items were then factor analyzed. Four factors were extracted and rotated orthogonally. Masie labeled the four factors as follows: "depression," "marital satisfaction," "optimism about the future," and "feelings of gender-role inadequacies." The factor scores on these four scales were analyzed in four separate (2 × 2) analyses of covariance, using the women's age and duration of the marriage as covariates. The following table summarizes the results of the statistical tests for the main and interaction effects (for each test there are 1 and 194 degrees of freedom):

	GENDER OF PARTNER (Male versus female)	**LOCUS OF FERTILITY PROBLEMS** (Self versus partner)	**GENDER × LOCUS INTERACTION**
Depression	$F = 5.9^*; p < .05$	$F = 6.7\dagger; p < .01$	$F = 3.9; p < 0.5$
Marital satisfaction	$F = 0.8$; ns	$F = 1.4; p < .05$	$F = 2.3$; ns
Optimism	$F = 1.9$; ns	$F = 2.1$; ns	$F = 1.5$; ns
Gender-role inadequacy	$F = 5.2^*; p < .05$	$F = 11.4\dagger; p < .001$	$F = 3.1$; ns

*Wife higher than husband
†Self higher than partner
ns, Not statistically significant.

Masie concluded that her hypotheses were partially supported by the data.

Review and critique this study with respect to the analysis of the data. To assist you in your critique, here are some guiding questions:

    a. For each variable in the study, what is the level of measurement?

    b. How many independent and dependent variables are there in this study?

    c. Considering responses to the above two questions and the size of the sample, did the researcher use the appropriate analysis? Suggest alternative ways to analyze the data and compare the information yielded in the two approaches.

    d. The test statistics shown are associated with a specific p level. Using the tables in the Appendix of the text, determine whether each p level is correct.

    e. What does each of the statistical tests signify?

2. Below are several suggested research articles. Read one of these articles, paying special attention to the analysis of the data. Respond to questions a through e from Question D.1. in terms of the actual research study.

- Appel, S. J., Harrell, J. S., & Deng, S. (2002). Racial and socioeconomic differences in risk factors for cardiovascular disease among Southern rural women. *Nursing Research, 51,* 140–147.
- Barroso, J., Carlson, J. R., & Meynell, J. (2003). Physiological and psychological markers associated with HIV-related fatigue. *Clinical Nursing Research, 12,* 49–68
- Duncan, S. M., Hyndman, K., Estabrooks, C. A., Hesketh, K., Humphrey, C. K., Wong, J. S., Acorn, S., & Giovannetti, P. (2001). Nurses' experience of violence in Alberta and British Columbia hospitals. *Canadian Journal of Nursing Research, 32,* 57–78.
- Guthrie, B. J., Young, A. M., Williams, D. R., Boyd, C. J., & Kintner, E. K. (2002). African American girls' smoking habits and day-to-day experiences with racial discrimination. *Nursing Research, 51,* 183–190.
- Heilemann, M. V., Lee, K. A., Kury, F. S. (2002). Strengths and vulnerabilities of women of Mexican descent in relation to depressive symptoms. *Nursing Research, 51,* 175–182.

E. Special Projects

1. On the following page is a rotated factor matrix for a set of 20 Likert items administered to 300 teenagers in a study of teenage sexuality and contraceptive practices.

Using this matrix, do the following:

    a. Identify and label the underlying dimensions.

    b. Select the items that will form three scales.

    c. Compute factor scores for three individuals whose responses to the 20 items are as follows:

Mary: 1 2 5 3 5 4 2 3 4 4 3 1 1 4 2 1 4 1 2 4

Tom: 4 1 2 4 1 2 5 4 1 3 1 2 4 2 1 3 4 5 2 3

Debbie: 2 4 1 2 2 1 5 1 2 4 4 5 2 2 5 1 1 4 5 4

2. Design and describe a study in which you would use both factor analysis and discriminant function analysis.
3. Design and describe a study in which you would use life table analysis.

	Factor I	Factor II	Factor III
1. It is primarily the woman's responsibility to use birth control.	.10	.62	.22
2. It is difficult to talk to your boyfriend about what kind of birth control the two of you should use.	.09	−.07	.36
3. It can be exciting to take a chance on getting pregnant.	.72	−.03	.08
4. It is relatively easy to put the worry about pregnancy out of one's mind.	.18	−.02	.25
5. It is sometimes important to prove your love by taking a chance.	.48	−.21	.13
6. No form of birth control really works.	.18	.06	−.18
7. People are foolish to depend on luck when it comes to pregnancy risk.	−.40	.17	−.23
8. Every teen who really wants to use birth control can easily do so.	.16	−.02	−.47
9. Sometimes making love with a particular person is worth the chance of pregnancy.	.51	.11	−.12
10. The best birth control methods are those that the man uses.	−.09	−.42	.17
11. A woman sometimes has a really hard time avoiding sexual involvement even when there isn't any birth control available.	.05	−.04	.32
12. The problem with some birth control is that you have to plan for the possibility of intercourse ahead of time.	−.04	.03	.52
13. A woman can't really trust a man to handle contraception.	−.01	.39	.07
14. If you really love someone, the chances of pregnancy aren't so important.	.36	.12	−.01
15. Getting hold of good birth control is a lot of effort and bother.	.02	−.09	.61
16. A woman needs to be in control of birth control for her own protection.	.03	.43	−.15
17. It's pretty easy to protect oneself against a pregnancy.	−.11	.06	−.68
18. Having unprotected sex isn't worth the risk of disrupting your life.	−.58	−.07	.24
19. It's really a hassle to use birth control.	.22	−.01	.49
20. It's a man's duty to see that his partner is protected.	.08	−.47	−.20

CHAPTER **22**

Designing and Implementing a Quantitative Analysis Strategy

A. Matching Exercises

Match each phrase from Set B with one (or more) of the missing values strategies listed in Set A. Indicate the letter(s) corresponding to your response next to each of the statements in Set B.

SET A
a. Listwise deletion
b. Deletion of variable
c. Mean substitution
d. Estimation of missing value
e. Pairwise deletion

SET B   **RESPONSE**

1. Complete deletion of missing cases   _____
2. Results in a nonrectangular matrix   _____
3. Multiple regression can be used to achieve this   _____
4. Useful when there are missing values for a few items on a
   scale   _____
5. Not an attractive option when the missing values are on a
   key variable   _____
6. Not an attractive option when the sample size is very small   _____
7. Usually more precise than mean substitution   _____

8. A good solution if a study participant has extensive missing data   _____

9. Results in a sample that is a "moving target"   _____

10. Useful when there are missing data on a variable for a high percentage of study participants   _____

B. Completion Exercises

Write the words or phrases that correctly complete the following sentences.

1. Coding of research data for statistical analysis should ideally involve _____ symbols.

2. Variables measured on the _____ scale can be assigned an arbitrary code.

3. Variables that are inherently _____ do not need to be coded.

4. Closed-ended questions can usually be _____ .

5. In coding open-ended or unstructured materials, the coding categories should be mutually exclusive and _____ .

6. "Don't knows" and refusals are usually treated as _____ .

7. Each individual case (e.g., each study participant) in a study should be assigned a unique _____ .

8. _____ procedures are recommended to detect errors in data entry.

9. Entered data are not ready for analysis until they have been _____ .

10. Coding and data entry decisions should be fully _____ .

11. It is almost inevitable for a data set to have some _____, creating potential problems that the researcher must address.

12. If men had significantly more missing information than women on a question about their use of illegal drugs, this would indicate the presence of _____ .

13. If a data set had data values for all study participants on all variables, the data set would be a _____ of data.

14. Raw data often need to be _____ or altered before proceeding to statistical analysis.

15. When an item on a seven-point scale is changed from a value of 2 to a value of 6, this is called a(n) _____ .

16. Researchers collecting data from several sites often perform tests to determine if the data can be _____ .

17. When data are voluminous, researchers sometimes develop _____ to guide the analysis of data.

18. In quantitative studies, the statistical analyses yield the _____of the study.

19. The first step in the interpretation of research findings involves a scrutiny of the _____ of the results, based on various types of evidence.

20. It is useful for a researcher to perform a _____when results relating to the main hypothesis tests are not statistically significant.

21. In quantitative analysis, the results are generally in the form of _____ and _____.

22. Interpretation of results is easiest when the results are consistent with the researcher's _____ .

23. Because researchers are not generally interested in discovering relationships exclusively for the research sample, an important part of the interpretive process involves an assessment of the _____ of the results.

24. An important research precept is that _____does not prove causation.

25. Nonsignificant findings mean that the null hypothesis is _____ _____ and significant findings mean that the null hypothesis is _____ .

C. Study Questions

1. Define the following terms. Compare your definition with the definition in Chapter 22 or in the glossary of the textbook.

   a. Data set: _____

   _____

   b. Coding: _____

   _____

   c. Missing values: _____

   _____

   d. Outlier: _____

   _____

   e. Wild code: _____

   _____

   f. Consistency check: _____

   _____

   g. Listwise deletion: _____

   _____

   h. Pairwise deletion: _____

   _____

   i. Ceiling effect: _____

   _____

   j. Manipulation check: _____

   _____

   k. Cohort effect: _____

   _____

   l. Negative results: _____

   _____

   m. Positive results: _____

   _____

n. Mixed results: _____

_____

2. Create a table shell for displaying some statistical analyses using the data presented in Exercise E.1 in Chapter 19 of this study guide.

3. Below is a research article in which the researchers obtained mixed results— that is, some hypotheses were supported, and others were not. Review and critique the researchers' interpretation of the findings and suggest some possible alternatives.

> Svavarsdottir, E. K., McCubbin, M. A., & Kane, J. H. (2000). Well-being of parents of young children with asthma. *Research in Nursing & Health, 23,* 346–358.

D. Application Exercise

1. Here is a summary of a fictitious study. Read the summary and then respond to the questions that follow:

> Armstrong and Kunstler (2003) studied the relationship between marital quality during pregnancy and postpartum depression in a sample of couples expecting their first child. Data on marital satisfaction, perceived relationship quality, and egalitarianism of marital roles were gathered during the second trimester of the pregnancy from 157 couples (157 women and 116 men completed three scales and demographic forms). Information on birth outcomes were available for 149 infants. Maternal depression was measured 2 weeks after delivery for 138 mothers. Here are some of the things that the researchers decided to do before they conducted their substantive analyses:
>
> • Use data for only the 110 families for which data for all three types of information were available (male and female partners' marital data; birth outcomes; and maternal depression).
> • Compute the reliability (internal consistency) of the three marital quality scales separately for men and women.
> • Analyze differences between the men who did and did not complete the predelivery information (in terms of their partner's background characteristics and perceptions of marital quality).
> • Analyze differences between the women who agreed to complete the depression scale postpartum and those who did not (in terms of own and their partner's background characteristics and perceptions of marital quality, and birth outcomes).

Review and comment on these decisions. Suggest alternative and additional preanalysis activities for the researchers. To aid you in this task, here are some guiding questions:

   a. Did the researchers handle missing values problems in the most effective manner? What other approaches might have been used? What are the consequences of the alternative strategies?

   b. How did the researchers evaluate data quality? Was this an appropriate strategy? What other steps could have been taken to ensure high-quality data?

   c. What did the researchers do to evaluate bias? Was this an appropriate strategy? What other methods could have been used to examine bias?

   d. What (if any) additional analyses should the researchers have undertaken before addressing the main substantive analyses?

2. Below are several suggested research articles. Read one of these articles and respond (to the extent possible) to questions a through d from Question D.1 with regard to this actual research study.

- Buist, A., Morse, C. A., & Durkin, S. (2003). Men's adjustment to fatherhood: Implications for obstetric health care. *Journal of Obstetric, Gynecologic, and Neonatal Nursing, 32,* 172–180.

- Leinonen, T., Leino-Kilpi, H., Stahlberg, M., & Lertola, K. (2003). Comparing patient and nurse perceptions of perioperative care quality. *Applied Nursing Research, 16,* 29–37.

- Lindeke, L. L., Stanley, J. R., Else, B. S., & Mills, M.M. (2002). Neonatal predictors of school-based services used by NICU graduates at school age. *MCN: The Journal of Maternal/Child Nursing, 27,* 41–46.

- McCullagh, M., Lusk, S. L., & Ronis, D. L. (2002). Factors influencing use of hearing protection among farmers. *Nursing Research, 51,* 33–40.

E. Special Projects

1. Read one of the studies listed in Question D.3 of this chapter. Compare your interpretation of the results with the interpretation of the researchers, as presented in the Discussion section of the report.

2. Based on the table presented in Question D.1 of Chapter 20 of this study guide, prepare a written discussion of the results of Pfeil's study.

CHAPTER **23**

Analyzing Qualitative Data

A. Matching Exercises

Match each descriptive statement from Set B with one or more types of qualitative analyses from Set A. Indicate the letter(s) corresponding to your response next to each item in Set B.

SET A
a. Grounded theory analysis
b. Phenomenological analysis
c. Ethnographic analysis
d. None of the above

SET B   **RESPONSE**

1. Involves the development of coding categories   _____

2. Begins with "open coding"   _____

3. One method of analysis was developed by Colaizzi   _____

4. Data can be organized using computer software   _____

5. One method of analysis was developed by Glaser & Strauss   _____

6. May involve the development of a taxonomy   _____

7. Involves the use of a metamatrix   _____

8. Often uses a style most likely to be described as "template analysis style"   _____

9. Often uses a style most likely to be described as "editing analysis style"   _____

10. Requires the use of quasi-statistics   _____

B. Completion Exercises

Write the words or phrases that correctly complete the following sentences.

1. Data collection and data analysis typically occur _____ in qualitative studies, not as separate phases.

2. The four processes that play a role in qualitative analysis are _____ _____, _____, _____, and _____.

3. The main task in organizing qualitative data involves the development of a method of _____ and _____ the data.

4. A _____ is a physical file that is organized to contain all material relating to a topic area.

5. Traditional methods of organizing qualitative data are being replaced by _____.

6. The analysis of qualitative data generally begins with a search for _____ .

7. In grounded theory, the process of breaking down the data, examining them, and comparing them to other segments is referred to as _____ _____.

8. In a grounded theory study, the initial phase of coding is referred to as _____.

9. In grounded theory studies, coding of information relating only to the core variable is referred to as _____ coding.

10. A particular type of core variable in a grounded theory study is the _____ or BSP.

11. The concept of _____ involves finding a convergence between what is in the data and preexisting categories from earlier work.

12. An alternative approach to Glaser and Strauss's approach to grounded theory analysis was developed by _____.

13. Colaizzi, Giorgi, and VanKaam's methods of analysis are used to analyze data from a study within the _____ tradition.

14. One of Van Manen's approaches to data analysis is referred to as the _____ approach, which involves an analysis of every sentence of data.

15. The four levels of analysis in Spradley's ethnographic method are _____ analysis, _____ analysis, _____ analysis, and _____ analysis.

16. The use of _____ involves an accounting of the frequency with which certain themes and relationships are supported by the data.

C. Study Questions

1. Define the following terms. Compare your definition with the definition in Chapter 23 or in the glossary of the textbook.

   a. Qualitative analysis: _____

   _____

   b. Categorization scheme: _____

   _____

   c. Theme: _____

   _____

   d. Conceptual files: _____

   _____

   e. Memos: _____

   _____

   f. Fit: _____

   _____

   g. Open coding: _____

   _____

   h. Selective coding: _____

   _____

   i. Core category: _____

   _____

   j. Duquesne school: _____

   _____

   k. Utrecht school: _____

   _____

   l. Domain analysis:_____

   _____

   m. Taxonomic analysis: _____

   _____

   n. Metamatrix: _____

   _____

2. For each of the research questions below, indicate whether you think a researcher should collect primarily qualitative or quantitative data. Justify your response.

   a. How do victims of AIDS cope with the discovery of their illness?_____

   _____

   b. What important dimensions of nursing practice differ in developed and underdeveloped countries? _____

   _____

   c. What is the effect of therapeutic touch on patient well-being?_____

   _____

   d. Do nurse practitioners and physicians differ in the performance of triage functions?_____

   _____

   e. Is a patient's length of stay in a hospital related to the quality or quantity of his or her social supports?_____

   _____

   f. How does the typical American feel about such new reproductive technologies as in vitro fertilization?_____

   _____

   g. What are the psychological consequences of having an organ transplantation?

   _____

   h. By what processes do women make decisions about having amniocentesis?

   _____

i. What factors are most predictive of a woman giving birth to a very-low-birth-weight infant? _____

_____

j. What effects does caffeine have on gastrointestinal motility? _____

_____

3. A category scheme for coding interviews with recently divorced women follows.

CODING SCHEME FOR STUDY
OF ADJUSTMENT TO DIVORCE

1. Divorce-related issues
   a. Adjustment to divorce
   b. Divorce-induced problems
   c. Advantages of divorce
2. General psychologic state
   a. Before divorce
   b. During divorce
   c. Current
3. Physical health
   a. Before divorce
   b. During divorce
   c. Current
4. Relationship with children
   a. General quality
   b. Communication
   c. Shared activities
   d. Structure of relationship
5. Parenting
   a. Discipline and child-rearing
   b. Feelings about parenthood
   c. Feelings, about single parenthood
6. Friendship/social participation
   a. Dating and marriage,
   b. Friendships
   c. Social groups, leisure
   d. Social support
7. Employment/education
   a. Employment experiences
   b. Educational experiences
   c. Job and career goals
   d. Educational goals
8. Workload
   a. Coping with workload
   b. Schedule
   c. Child care arrangements
9. Finances

Read the following excerpt, taken from a real interview. Use the coding scheme to code the topics discussed in this excerpt.

> I think raising the children is so much easier without the father around. There isn't two people conflicting back and forth. You know, like . . . like you discipline them during the day. They do something wrong, you're not saying, "When daddy gets home, you're going to get a spanking." You know, you do that. The kid gets a spanking right then and there. But when two people live together, they have their ways of raising and you have your ways of raising the children and it's so hard for two people to raise children. It's so much easier for one person. The only reason a male would be around is financial-wise. But me and the kids are happier now, and we get along with each other better, cause like, there isn't this competitive thing. My husband always wanted all the attention around here.

D. Application Exercises

1. Here is a brief summary of a fictitious qualitative study. Read the summary and then respond to the questions that follow.

   > Dolen (2003) studied the phenomenon of "being on precautions" from the perspective of hospitalized adults. She began her study, after securing authorization, by spending 2 days on the hospital units where data would be collected. The 2 days were spent familiarizing herself with the units, learning how best to collect the data, determining where she could position herself in an unobtrusive manner, and establishing a trusting relationship with the nursing staff.
   >
   > The data for the study were collected using observations and unstructured interviewing. Dolen selectively sampled all times of the day and all days of the week in 2-hour segments to make her observations. The time schedule began on a Monday morning at 7:00 AM and continued until 9:00 AM. On Tuesday, the observation time became 9:00 AM until 11:00 AM. Observations continued around the clock on consecutive days until no new information was being collected. Dolen either positioned herself directly outside the door to the patient's room or sat in the patient's room to make her observations. Observations included any activity or interaction between the patient and hospital staff or between the patient and Dolen. Unstructured interviewing involved asking patients to clarify why they were doing certain things and what they liked or disliked about the hospital experience.
   >
   > Dolen recorded the observations and data from the interviews in a log immediately after each 2-hour observation segment. All data were recorded in chronologic order. Dolen also recorded any feelings she had during the observation experience. As time progressed, she reread her field notes after every 4 hours of observation. As commonalities began to emerge from the data, she developed another section to her field notes according to similarity of content and referenced the daily log notes according to commonalities. Dolen continued making observations until she thought she had a "good feel for the data" and that additional observations or interactions would provide only redundant information. Five patients were observed.
   >
   > Categories that emerged from the data were labeled "avoidance," "devaluation as a person," and "loneliness." Evidence for the avoidance perspective came from patient

comments during informal conversations with the researcher and the observational field notes. The evidence included statements such as, "Nurses seldom come into the room because they have to put all that [pointing to precaution gowns] stuff on." "Look, she [the cleaning woman] won't come in the room. She's afraid of me." "Did you see that? Only my doctor would touch me. The rest were afraid to touch me." Observational field notes contained several notations of nurses coming to the door of the room asking, "Do you want anything?" but not entering the room.

The category "devaluation as a person" emerged from comments such as, "I don't like being treated as a specimen." "Do you have to wear gloves every time you take care of me [made to a nurse]?" "If I go to the door of the room, they [the nurses] yell at me [made to the researcher]."

The category "loneliness" was developed from field notes that observed patients occasionally putting the call light on to find out what time it was or how long until lunch, or asking about a noise they had heard. Comments that conveyed the same feeling of loneliness were, "Being confined in this room is like being in jail." "I can't wait to get out of here and have dinner with my friends." "The hours seem endless here."

Review and critique this study. Suggest alternative ways of collecting and analyzing the data for the research problem. To assist you in your critique, here are some guiding questions:

a. Comment on the choice of research approach. Was a qualitative research approach suitable for the phenomenon being studied? In your opinion, would a more quantitative research approach have been more appropriate?

b. The data in the study were collected by observation and informal interviewing. Could the data have been collected in another way? Should they have been?

c. The researcher recorded her observations, feelings, and interviews immediately after each 2-hour observation period. Comment on the appropriateness of this method. Can you identify any biases that could be present in this choice of method? Suggest alternative ways of recording the data.

d. Categorize the field notes made in the study according to their purpose. What additional types of field notes would you have included?

e. How did the researcher handle the concept of theoretical saturation? Could you recommend any improvements?

f. What types of validation procedures did the researcher use? Can you suggest additional procedures that might have improved the study?

g. Comment on the categories that emerged from the data. Do they appear to reflect accurately the data that were collected? Would you have developed different ones?

2. Below are several suggested research articles. Skim one or more of these articles and respond to questions a through g from Question D.1, to the extent possible, in terms of the actual research study.

- Clark, L. (2002). Mexican-origin mothers' experiences suing children's health care services. *Western Journal of Nursing Research, 24,* 159–179.

- Ehrmin, J. T. (2002). "That feeling of not feeling": Numbing the pain for substance-dependent African American women. *Qualitative Health Research, 12,* 780–791.
- Martell, L. K. (2001). Heading toward the new normal: A contemporary postpartum experience. *Journal of Obstetric, Gynecologic, and Neonatal Nursing, 30,* 496–596.
- Mercado-Martinez, F. J., & Ramos-Herrera, I. M. (2002). Diabetes: The layperson's theories of causality. *Qualitative Health Research, 12,* 792–806.
- Sword, W. (2003). Prenatal care use among women of low income: A matter of "taking care of self." *Qualitative Health Research, 13,* 319–332.

3. Below is a brief description of the data analysis in a fictitious qualitative study, followed by a critique. Do you agree with this critique? Can you add other comments relevant to the data analysis in this study?

Fictitious Study. Mastrianni (2003) was interested in learning about the health policies and health environments of child care centers. She began her study by spending a week in an urban day care center that provided child care services to children aged 10 weeks to preschool-age. The purpose of this preliminary step was to ascertain likely sources of information and to familiarize herself with the routine of child care environments.

The data for the study were collected through unstructured interviews with child care staff, through observation of activities during normal operating hours, and through the gathering of formal health policy statements from the administrators of the centers. The interviews with the staff focused on how staff handled illnesses among the children, what the patterns of illnesses were, how parents were notified in the case of a midday illness, to what extent medications were administered by the staff, and how the staff interpreted center policies relating to the admission of unwell children. Data were collected from 10 child care centers that served 20 or more children whose ages ranged from infant to preschool-age. A total of 68 staff interviews were completed.

Mastrianni's field notes from the observations and the interviews were transcribed and coded according to a coding scheme that evolved during the actual collection of data. Three major themes emerged from the data analysis. These were labeled uncertainty, conflict, and frustration. The types of evidence that gave rise to the uncertainty category included statements made by staff, such as: "I'm really not a very good judge of just where to draw the line in deciding whether to keep a child here or send her home." "I can't really remember what our health policies say on that." "I don't really know what the major health problems are among our kids—when they're absent, I just have one less kid to worry about."

Evidence of the conflict dimension included the researcher's observation that staff and parents sometimes had disagreements about whether a child was not well enough to attend. Also, staff made such statements as: "Health is a problem in child care centers because, on the one hand, allowing a sick kid to attend means that we'll have a lot of sick kids, but on the other hand, it's really tough on parents when their child care arrangements fall apart."

The category of frustration emerged from such statements as: "It's difficult to plan activities because absenteeism for health reasons is such a problem right now." "I can't seem to get the kids interested in thinking about good health or good nutrition—their parents are just as bad."

Mastrianni analyzed the data herself but shared preliminary results of her analyses with one of the directors of a child care center, who concurred with the thematic analysis. Mastrianni's analysis revealed that centers that had a formal arrangement with a health care provider were less likely to have staff who were uncertain. Conflict was a fairly universal theme but appeared to be more prevalent among those centers that served predominantly low-income families. Frustration was most likely to be observed and expressed among staff caring for older children.

Critique. Given Mastrianni's broad area of interest in health issues within child care centers, it seems appropriate that she conducted an in-depth, multifaceted qualitative study. The use of three complementary sources of data strengthened her study because it provided an opportunity for validating findings. At least from the brief description presented, however, it does not appear that these data sources were fully exploited. For example, no use appears to have been made of the written policy statements.

It appears that the author did little to validate the subjective thematic analysis. The analysis would have been greatly strengthened if Mastrianni had involved another investigator in the coding and analysis, if she had systematically searched for contrary evidence regarding the important themes, or if there had been an iterative approach in the analysis to check emerging themes against the data. Although it is laudable that Mastrianni invited comments from one of the child care center's directors, it is unfortunate that only one person's opinion was sought.

The true validity of Mastrianni's thematic analysis is difficult to evaluate without actually inspecting the data, but the brief description does not provide persuasive evidence that the analysis was thorough and unbiased. The data sources should have yielded a wealth of information about various aspects of the health policies and practices of the day care centers. Yet all three themes focus on the staff's feelings, and in all three cases these are negative feelings. What about their actions? What about their levels of competence in dealing with health issues? What about their sensitivity to the needs of their clients? It would appear that several of the excerpts included in support of Mastrianni's thematic analysis could have been conceptualized in a different way, suggesting that perhaps Mastrianni had some preconceived notions about what the unstructured interviews and observations would yield. It is possible that a reconceptualization (i.e., a thematic analysis of the same materials by a different investigator) could alter our impression of the health practices and policies of child care centers.

E. Special Projects

1. Get 10 or so people to write one or two paragraphs on their feelings about death and dying. Perform a thematic analysis of these paragraphs.

2. Read one of the studies listed in the "Studies Cited" section of Chapter 23 in the textbook. Generate several hypotheses that could be tested based on the reported findings.

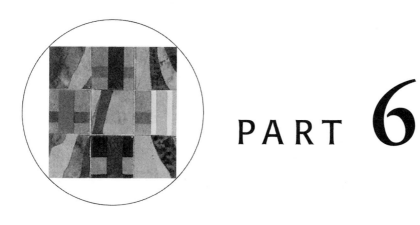

PART **6**

Communicating Research

CHAPTER **24**

Summarizing and Sharing Research Findings

A. Matching Exercises

Match each sentence from Set B with one of the sections in a research report in which these sentences would appear, as listed in Set A. Indicate the letter corresponding to your response next to each of the statements in Set B.

SET A
a. Introduction
b. Method section
c. Results section
d. Discussion section

SET B   RESPONSE

1. This study sought to understand how chronic recidivists to alcohol treatment programs define and experience their treatment.   _____

2. The sample consisted of 250 men aged 75 to 85 years, selected at random from 5 nursing homes.   _____

3. These findings suggest that nurses have become increasingly less accepting of traditional sex-role stereotypes.   _____

4. It is hypothesized that male and female paraplegics differ in their perceptions of the importance of architectural barriers.   _____

5. The 100 subjects were randomly assigned to the experimental and control groups using a random-numbers table.   _____

6. A central feature of the adaptation process is *coming to terms*, as exemplified by the following: "You learn that you will never again be able to do what you could do before, but you survive."   _____

7. A major flaw of studies conducted to date is the low reliability of the instruments the researchers used.   _____

8. The findings reported here are consistent with the work of Gardner (2001) and Schoen (2002).   _____

9. Age at marriage was found to be significantly related to both educational attainment ($r = -.25$) and number of children ($r = -.38$).   _____

10. Informants were selected on the basis of theoretical needs emerging during the course of data collection.   _____

B. Completion Exercises

Write the words or phrases that correctly complete the sentences below.

1. At professional conferences, an alternative to presenting a paper orally in front of an audience is to present findings at a _____.

2. An unpublished research report submitted for publication is usually referred to as a _____.

3. The person who has overall responsibility for a research report submitted for publication is called the _____.

4. The conventional format for organizing quantitative research reports is referred to as the _____ format.

5. The _____ section of a report discusses the researcher's aims, the research questions, and the context of the study.

6. The _____ section of a report describes what the researcher did to gather and analyze the data.

7. Research findings are described in the _____section of a report.

8. Statistical information can most effectively and succinctly be displayed in _____ .

9. Graphic presentations of statistical information are usually referred to as
_____ .

10. Interpretations   of   results   are   normally   presented   in   the
_____ section of a report.

11. The   main   communication   outlet   for   scholarly   research   activity   is
_____ .

12. When a research report is authored by more than one person who made equal
contributions, the names are listed _____ .

C. Study Questions

1. Define the following terms. Compare your definition with the definition in
Chapter 24 of the textbook or in the glossary.

a. Research report: _____

_____

b. Front matter: _____

_____

c. Paper format thesis: _____

_____

d. Query letter: _____

_____

e. Corresponding author: _____

_____

f. Blind review: _____

_____

g. Call for papers: _____

_____

h. Poster session: _____

_____

i. Refereed journal: _____

_____

  j. ejournal: _____

  _____

2. The following sentences all have stylistic flaws. Suggest ways in which the sentences could be improved.

  a. ICU nurses experience more stress than nurses on a general ward ($t = 2.5$, $df = 148$, $p < .05$)

  _____

  _____

  b. "A Study Investigating the Effect of Primary Care Nursing on the Emotional Well-Being of Patients in a Cardiac Care Unit."

  _____

  _____

  c. The nonsignificant results demonstrate that there is no relationship between diet and hyperkinesis.

  _____

  _____

  d. It has, therefore, been proved that people have a more negative body image if the age of onset of obesity is before age 20 years.

  _____

  _____

  e. The positive, significant relationship indicates that occupational stress causes sleep disturbances.

  _____

  _____

3. Suppose that you were the author of a research article with the titles indicated below. For each, name two different journals to which your article could be submitted for publication.

  a. "Parental attachment to children with Down's syndrome."
  b. "Sexual functioning among the elderly: The lived experience of noninstitutionalized men and women in their 70s."
  c. "Comparison of therapists' and clients' expectations regarding psychiatric therapy."
  d. "The effects of fetal monitoring on selected birth outcomes."
  e. "Effectiveness of alternative methods of relieving pressure sores."

4. Suppose you were studying the psychological well-being of women who had just experienced a miscarriage in comparison of women who were still pregnant in the second month of their pregnancy. For these two groups, the mean scores, respectively, on four scales are 15.1 and 10.7 (depression); 23.6 and 23.9 (mood); 17.9 and 15.7 (marital satisfaction); and 18.9 and 25.8 (self-efficacy). Prepare a table to display these results. (Embellish the table by inventing either standard deviation information or results of *t*-tests).

D. Application Exercises

1. Below is a description of a fictitious study. Read the summary and then respond to the questions that follow.

> Lavine and Wyse (2003) hypothesized that preschool children from single-parent families are more likely than those from two-parent families to display negative behavioral and psychosocial patterns. They administered a behavioral checklist to 30 divorced mothers and 30 married mothers who accompanied their preschool child (3–5 years of age) during immunization for measles. Each mother was asked to indicate the frequency with which these preschool children exhibited a series of behaviors ("very often," "fairly often," "sometimes," or "never"). Examples of the behavioral items include, "often cries with little or no apparent reason," "tends to sulk when unable to have his or her own way," and "has trouble making or keeping friends." The items were combined to form three subscales: Home and Family; Friends and Peers; and General Behaviors. Overall Behavioral Adjustment scores were also computed. The table below presents the results:

| | ONE-PARENT | TWO-PARENT | | |
	Means*	*Means**	*t*	*p*
Home and Family	17.5	16.8	1.5	> .05
Friends and Peers	19.1	19.4	0.9	> 0.5
General Behaviors	24.7	25.3	1.1	> 0.5
Overall Behavioral Adjustment	61.3	61.5	0.7	> 0.5

*Higher scores reflect *better* adjustment.

Here is how Lavine and Wyse described their results:

> Contrary to expectations, the behavioral patterns of the children from intact and one-parent homes were very similar. With respect to Home and Family behaviors, in fact, children in the one-parent homes were superior. Friendship patterns and interactions with peers were virtually identical in the two groups. In terms of general behaviors, such as crying, pouting, or acting out, the children from the two-parent families showed a slight edge. Overall, the two groups performed about equivalently. Thus, it may be concluded that preschool children who live in one-parent families are not handicapped by the absence of their fathers. Their behaviors are normal and not dif-

ferent from those of their same-aged peers from intact homes. In one area, children from the one-parent home show evidence of more favorable behaviors than those with both parents at home.

Review and critique the above description. Suggest alternative ways of describing and interpreting the results. To help you in your critique, here are some guiding questions:

    a. Comment on the content of the excerpt. Did the author omit discussing any important results? Was there any redundancy—could the summary have been more succinct?

    b. Comment on the accuracy of the report. Does the text agree with the table? Does the report imply statistically significant results that were in fact not in the data?

    c. Comment on the style of the report. Do the authors use language that is too subjective? Do they fail to use language that is in keeping with the tentative nature of research? Do the authors use jargon or unnecessary technical terms?

    d. Comment on the authors' interpretation of the results. Do they read too much into the data? Do the authors suggest several possible explanations for the findings? In the interpretation, do the author try to take into consideration such factors as the smallness of the sample, the influence of extraneous variables, inadequacies of the measuring instrument, and so on?

2. Below are several suggested research articles. Skim one (or more) of these articles, focusing especially on the researcher's results and discussion sections. Respond to questions a through d from Question D.1 in terms of the actual research study.

- Baumann, L. C., Chang, M., & Hoebeke, R. (2002). Clinical outcomes for low-income adults with hypertension and diabetes. *Nursing Research, 51*, 191–198.
- Davis, R. E. (2002). Leave-taking experiences in the lives of abused women. *Clinical Nursing Research, 11*, 285–305.
- Funk, M., Ostfeld, A. M., Chang, V. M., & Lee,R. A. (2002). Racial differences in the use of cardiac procedures in patients with acute myocardial infarction. *Nursing Research, 51*, 148–157.
- Gingrich, P. M., & Fogel, C. I. (2003). Herbal therapy use by perimenopausal women. Journal of *Obsteteric, Gynecologic, and Neonatal Nursing, 32*, 181–189.
- Kolanowski, A. M., Litaker, M. S., & Baumann, M. A. (2002). Theory-based intervention for dementia behaviors: A within-person analysis over time. *Applied Nursing Research, 15*, 87–96.
- Wood, F. G. (2002). Ethnic differences in exercise among adults with diabetes. *Western Journal of Nursing Research, 24*, 502–515.

E. Special Projects

1. Suppose that you were studying maternal behavior in mothers of normal and handicapped children. Fifty mothers from each group are observed interacting with their children (7–10 years of age) in a laboratory setting for 30 minutes. Some data are presented below:

MEAN NO. OF:	MOTHERS WITH NORMAL CHILDREN	MOTHERS WITH HANDICAPPED CHILDREN	*t*
Times mother initiates conversations	10.2	12.8	2.3
Minutes of silence	14.9	13.8	1.7
Times mother laughs or smiles	8.4	7.9	1.2
Direct maternal commands	8.7	6.1	3.8
Encouraging or supportive comments	4.1	5.7	2.4

Write a brief Results and Discussion section for these data.

2. Read the article, "Advance directives and community-dwelling older adults, " by Hamel, Guse, Hawrank, and Bond, which appeared in *Western Journal of Nursing Research* (2002), volume 31, pages 143–158. This article has a traditional style of abstract (i.e., a 1-paragraph summary). Rewrite the abstract, using the "new style" of abstract such as that used in the journal *Nursing Research* (i.e., with the following subsections: Background, Objectives, Methods, Results, and Conclusions).

3. Suggest titles for five of the fictitious studies described in the Application sections of this study guide.

CHAPTER **25**

Writing a Research Proposal

A. Matching Exercises

Match each statement designating a section of a National Institutes of Health grant application from Set B with one (or more) of the phrases listed in Set A. Indicate the letter(s) corresponding to your response next to each of the statements in Set B.

SET A
a. Specific aims section
b. Background and significance section
c. Preliminary studies section
d. Research design and methods section
e. None of these sections

SET B   **RESPONSE**

1. Includes the budget   _____

2. Includes a review of previous research   _____

3. Includes a summary of the study objectives   _____

4. Should be no more than three pages   _____

5. Includes a description of the proposed sample   _____

6. Allows the investigators to elaborate their research qualifications   _____

7. Includes rationales for methodologic decisions   _____

8. Has a recommended page limitation of one page   _____

9. May include the work plan   _____

10. Has a recommended page limitation of eight pages   _____

B. Completion Exercises

Write the words or phrases that correctly complete the sentences below.

1. Proposals often begin with a brief synopsis or _____ of the proposed research.

2. The _____ describes the plan and schedule according to which project tasks would be accomplished.

3. The _____ translates the project activities into monetary terms.

4. A funding agency sometimes publicizes the _____ that will be used in making evaluative decisions about submitted proposals.

5. The set of skills involved in securing project funding is referred to as the _____ .

6. The basic NIH grant program is the _____.

7. The first part of the dual review system within NIH involves a _____ .

8. Applications to the Public Health Service that are approved for funding are assigned a _____.

9. Written critiques of grant applications through the NIH are provided on the _____ .

10. The two major types of federal disbursements are _____and _____.

11. RFP is an acronym for _____ .

12. RFA is an acronym for _____.

C. Study Questions

1. Define the following terms. Compare your definition with the definition in Chapter 25 or in the glossary of the textbook.

   a. Proposal: _____

   _____

    b. Work plan: _____

_____

    c. Front matter: _____

_____

    d. Program announcement: _____

_____

    e. Grant: _____

_____

    f. Contract:_____

_____

    g. R01 grant: _____

_____

    h. AREA award: _____

_____

    i. Direct costs:_____

_____

    j. Indirect costs: _____

_____

    k. Priority rating or score: _____

_____

    l. Study section: _____

_____

2. Chapter 25 of the text described several major sections of Public Health Service grant applications. In which sections would the following statements ordinarily be found?

    a. Study participants, who will include young adults who have been treated for a drug overdose, will initially be recruited through the emergency room of a local hospital. Network sampling will then be used to contact a broader population of those with an overdose experience.

_____

_____

b. The primary hypothesis is that paraplegics who receive pool therapy will perform better on tests of muscle strength than those who receive other types of exercise.

_____

_____

c. Dr. Hogan, who will direct the proposed research, has recently completed a 3-year longitudinal study of the coping mechanisms of parents with a Down syndrome infant.

_____

_____

d. The major threat to the internal validity of the proposed study is selection bias, which will be dealt with through the careful selection of comparison subjects and through statistical adjustment of preexisting differences.

_____

_____

e. All subjects will be asked to sign informed consent forms.

_____

_____

f. The proposed research will have the potential of restructuring the delivery of health care in rural areas.

_____

_____

D. Application Exercises

1. Below is a Specific Aims section from a grant application that was funded by the U.S. Office of Adolescent Pregnancy Programs.*

SPECIFIC AIMS
Substantial percentages of children in our society are born to young women who are teenagers. Despite the growth of interest in the "epidemic" of teenage pregnancy, relatively little attention has been paid to the parenting styles and behaviors of young

---

* Polit, "Parenting among low-income teenage mothers," awarded to Humanalysis, Inc. Reprinted with permission of Humanalysis, Inc.

mothers or to the development of their children, particularly in well-designed, longitudinal research.

The proposed research will use a combined observational/interview approach to collect information about the parental styles and attitudes, the family and home environment, and children's development in a sample of about 300 low-income young women who first became pregnant when they were 17 or younger, and whose oldest child is now about 5 years of age. Three rounds of interviews with these mothers have already been completed, in which extensive information about their backgrounds, economic circumstances, social support networks, household structure, psychological characteristics, and use of formal services (including parenting education) was gathered. The baseline interviews with these women, conducted either during their pregnancy or shortly after delivery, also measured parenting knowledge and perceived competence in parenting skills. The women in the sample reside in six geographically dispersed communities (Bedford-Stuyvesant, NY; Harlem, NY; Phoenix, AZ; San Antonio, TX; Riverside, CA; and Fresno, CA) and represent an ethnic mix of African-American, Hispanic, and white young mothers.

The longitudinal nature of this research will make it possible to test a comprehensive model of the effects of maternal age on several parenting and child development outcomes. The availability of extensive background information will also permit background influences (such as predelivery family structure and financial circumstances, early school experiences, educational aspirations, self-esteem, and family size expectations) to be controlled, yielding a more sensitive test of the hypothesized effects. In brief, the proposed research will examine the extent to which a teen mother's parenting knowledge is influenced by her age at first birth and her exposure to parenting education classes, net of other factors. Parenting behaviors (such as warmth, punitiveness, and stimulation of the child's learning) are hypothesized to be influenced by three major factors: characteristics of the mother (including her parenting knowledge), characteristics of the child, and contextual factors, such as stress and social support. Finally, the model predicts that child development outcomes (including cognitive development, social/behavioral adjustment, and physical health) are a function of parenting behaviors and the home environment, as well as characteristics of the child.

Review and critique this section of the grant application. To assist you in your critique, here are some guiding questions:

a. Is the presentation sufficiently specific? Does the author make overly general statements about what the research will accomplish?
b. Is the presentation clear and succinct? Is it direct and to the point?
c. Does the presentation sound convincing and authoritative? Does the researcher seem knowledgeable about the substantive issues?
d. Do the objectives sound manageable? That is, does it appear that the researcher will actually be able to accomplish her objectives, or is the scope of her objectives overly broad?

2. Information relating to a budget for a fictitious project is presented next:

A nurse researcher wanted to study student attrition among minority nursing school students. She proposed a critical incidents study of the experiences leading to minority students' decisions to drop out of their nursing programs. The study was to involve interviews with 150 minority dropouts in three states. Below is a tentative budget for such a project.

Budget: Minority Attrition Study

Personnel

Wasser (Principal Investigator)	40 weeks @ $1,500/wk	$60,000
Pehl (Interviewer)	10 weeks @ $600/wk	6,000
Licata (Interviewer)	10 weeks @ $600/wk	6,000
Gorss (Research Assistant)	15 weeks @ $400/wk	6,000
Castelot (Admin. Assistant)	26 weeks @ $450/wk	11,700
		$89,700
Fringe benefits @ 25%		22,425
TOTAL PERSONNEL		$112,125

Non personnel

Supplies $75/month x 12 months	$ 900
Xeroxing $75/month x 12 months	900
Printing questionnaires	600
Data entry 600 records x $1.00/record	600
Travel 3000 miles x $.365/mile	1,095
Statistical consultants 10 days @ $500/day	5,000
TOTAL NON PERSONNEL	$9,095

TOTAL DIRECT COSTS	**$121,220**

Review and comment on this budget in terms of the following:

a. The inclusion of all relevant budget categories for the proposed study.

b. Your perceptions of whether any given category is overbudgeted or under-budgeted.

E. Special Projects

1. Prepare a one-page Special Aims section for a research project you would like to conduct.

2. Identify at least one federal agency and two foundations that might be appropriate for sending a research proposal for a project in which you are interested.

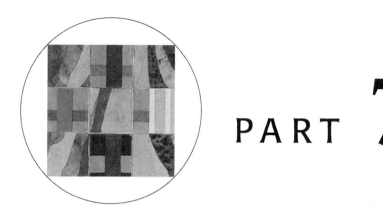

PART 7

Using Research
Results

CHAPTER **26**

Evaluating Research Reports

A. Matching Exercises

Match each of the questions in Set B with the research decision being evaluated, as listed in Set A. Indicate the letter corresponding to your response next to each of the statements in Set B.

SET A
a. Evaluating the research design decisions
b. Evaluating the population specification and sampling plan
c. Evaluating the data collection procedures
d. Evaluating the analytic decisions

SET B   **RESPONSE**

1. Was there a sufficient number of subjects?   _____

2. Was there evidence of adequate reliability and validity?   _____

3. Would a more limited specification have controlled some extraneous variables not covered by the research design?   _____

4. Would nonparametric tests have been more appropriate?   _____

5. Were respondents assured anonymity or confidentiality?   _____

6. Were threats to internal validity adequately controlled?   _____

7. Were the statistical tests appropriate, given the level of measurement of the variables?   _____

8. Were response-set biases minimized?   _____

9. Was the comparison group equivalent to the experimental group?   _____

10. Should the data have been collected prospectively?   _____

11. Were triangulation procedures used as a method of validation?   _____

12. Were constant comparison procedures appropriately used to refine relevant categories?   _____

13. Did the researcher stay in the field long enough to gain an emic perspective?   _____

14. Were informants asked to comment on the emerging themes?   _____

15. Was a phenomenological approach appropriate for the research question?   _____

B. Completion Exercises

Write the words or phrases that correctly complete the following sentences.

1. The research process involves numerous methodologic _____ _____, each of which could affect the quality of the study.

2. A good critique should identify both _____ and _____ of a study.

3. An evaluation of the relevance of a study to some aspect of the nursing profession involves critiquing the _____ dimension of a research study.

4. An evaluation of the researcher's plan to avoid self-selection biases involves critiquing the _____ dimension of a research study.

5. An evaluation of the way in which human subjects were treated involves critiquing the _____ dimension of a research study.

6. An evaluation of the sense the researcher tried to make of the results involves critiquing the _____ dimension of the research study.

7. An evaluation of the objectivity of the research report involves critiquing the _____ dimension of the research study.

C. Study Questions

1. Define the following terms. Compare your definitions with the definitions in Chapter 26 or in the glossary of the textbook.

   a. Critique: _____

   _____

   b. Research decisions: _____

   _____

   c. Methodologic dimension: _____

   _____

2. Read and critique one or more of the following articles (or other articles in the nursing research literature), and apply the questions in the boxes in Chapter 26 of the textbook. Prepare two to three pages of "bullet points" that indicate the major strengths and weaknesses of the study.

   - Clark, P. C. (2002). Effects of individual and family hardiness on caregiver depression and fatigue. *Research in Nursing & Health, 25,* 37–48.
   - Daggett, L. M. (2002). Living with loss: Middle-aged men face spousal bereavement. *Qualitative Health Research, 12,* 625–639.
   - Harrison, T., & Stuifbergen, A. (2002). Disability, social support, and concern for children: Depression in mothers with multiple sclerosis. *Journal of Obstetric, Gynecologic, and Neonatal Nursing, 31,* 444–453.
   - Resnick, B. (2002). Testing the effect of the WALC intervention on exercise adherence in older adults. *Journal of Gerontological Nursing, 28,* 40–49.
   - Rexilius, S. J., Mundt, C., Erickson-Megel, M., & Agrawal, S. (2002). Therapeutic effects of massage therapy and handling touch on caregivers of patients undergoing autologous hematopoietic stem cell transplant. *Oncology Nursing Forum, 29,* E35–44.
   - Rose, L., Mallinson, R. K., & Walton-Moss, B. (2002). A grounded theory study of families responding to mental illness. *Western Journal of Nursing Research, 24,* 516–536.
   - Werezak, L., & Stewart, N. (2002). Learning to live with early dementia. *Canadian Journal of Nursing Research, 34,* 67–85.

3. Read the following qualitative research report and identify the study's major strengths and limitations:

   Loeb, S. J., Penrod, J., Falkenstern, S., Gueldner, S. A., & Poon, L. W. (2003). Supporting older adults living with multiple chronic conditions. *Western Journal of Nursing Research, 25,* 8–29.

Now, read the two commentaries of the study that immediately follow the report (pages 23–27). Do any of your comments overlap with those of the commentators? Do you agree or disagree with either or both sets of comments?

D. Application Exercises

At the end of this study guide, in Part VII, are two actual research reports, one for a qualitative study and the other for a quantitative study. Read one or both of these reports, and prepare a three- to five-page critique summarizing the major strengths and weaknesses of the study.

E. Special Projects

1. Prepare a list of the 10 most important questions that would need to be addressed in a critique of the methodologic dimensions of a qualitative study.

2. Rewrite Nelson's report in Chapter 13 of Polit, Beck, and Hungler's (2001) *Study Guide to Accompany Essentials of Nursing Research,* (5th edition), pages 189–196, using some of the suggestions from the critique.

CHAPTER **27**

Utilizing Research: Putting Research Evidence Into Nursing Practice

A. Matching Exercises

Match each of the RU/EBP strategies from Set B with one of the roles indicated in Set A. Indicate the letter corresponding to your response for the most likely role(s) next to each of the strategies in Set B.

SET A
a. Nursing researchers
b. Nursing faculty and educators
c. Practicing nurses and nursing students
d. Nursing administrators

SET B   **RESPONSE**

1. Become involved in a journal club   _____
2. Perform replications   _____
3. Prepare integrative reviews of research literature   _____
4. Offer resources for RU or EBP projects   _____
5. Disseminate findings   _____
6. Specify clinical implications of findings   _____
7. Read research reports critically   _____
8. Foster intellectual curiosity in the work environment   _____
9. Provide a forum for communication between clinicians and researchers   _____
10. Expect evidence that a procedure is effective   _____

B. Completion Exercises

Write the words or phrases that correctly complete the following sentences.

1. _____ refers to the use of some aspect of a scientific investigation in an application unrelated to the original research.

2. There has been considerable concern about the _____ between knowledge production and knowledge utilization.

3. A prominent theory for modeling how knowledge gets disseminated and used is the _____.

4. The most well known nursing research utilization project, conducted in Michigan, is the _____ Project.

5. _____ begins with an empirically derived innovation that gets examine for possible adoption in practice; _____ begins with a search for how best to solve specific practice problems.

6. The _____ Collaboration is an international effort to integrate and disseminate evidence about effective health care practices.

7. A(n) _____ ranks studies according to the strength of evidence they provide.

8. A widely held view is that the strongest evidence for EBP comes from _____.

9. The _____ model provides guidance for an individual utilization or EBP effort.

10. In the Iowa Model of EBP, the two starting points for an organizational utilization project are referred to as _____ trigger and _____ trigger.

11. A typical method of assembling and evaluating evidence on a topic has been the preparation of a(n) _____.

12. Part of the RU/EBP process involves an assessment of the _____ of an innovation in a new practice setting (e.g., assessing transferability and feasibility, and computing a cost–benefit ratio).

13. Two methods of searching for prior research are the _____ approach (footnote chasing of cited studies) and the _____ approach (searching citations forward).

14. Meta-analysts sometimes conduct _____ analyses to determine whether the exclusion of low-quality studies alters the conclusions.

15. To deal with the issue of not including unpublished studies in meta-analyses, a _____ number is sometimes calculated to estimate the number of studies with nonsignificant results needed to reverse conclusions.

C. Study Questions

1. Define the following terms. Compare your definition with the definition in Chapter 27 or in the glossary of the textbook.

   a. Instrumental utilization: _____

   _____

   b. Conceptual utilization: _____

   _____

   c. Knowledge creep: _____

   _____

   d. Decision accretion: _____

   _____

   e. Awareness stage of adoption: _____

   _____

   f. Persuasion state of adoption: _____

   _____

   g. Problem-focused trigger: _____

   _____

   h. Knowledge-focused trigger: _____

   _____

   i. Evidence report: _____

   _____

    j. Metasynthesis: _____

    _____

    k. Voting methods: _____

    _____

2. Think about a nursing procedure that you have learned. What is the basis for this procedure? Determine whether the procedure is based on scientific evidence indicating that the procedure is effective. If it is not based on scientific evidence, on what is it based, and why do you think scientific evidence was not used?

3. Identify the factors in your own practice setting that you think facilitate or inhibit research utilization and evidence-based practice (or, in an educational setting, the factors that promote or inhibit a climate in which RU/EBP is valued).

4. Read either Brett's (1987) article regarding the adoption of 14 nursing innovations ("Use of nursing practice research findings," *Nursing Research, 36,* pp. 344–349) or the more recent (1990) replication study based on the same 14 innovations by Coyle and Sokop ("Innovation adoption behavior among nurses," *Nursing Research, 39,* pp. 176–180). For each of the 14 innovations, indicate whether you are aware of the findings, persuaded that the findings should be used, use the findings sometimes in a clinical situation, or use the findings always in a clinical situation.

    1. _____

    2. _____

    3. _____

    4. _____

    5. _____

    6. _____

    7. _____

    8. _____

    9. _____

  10. _____

  11. _____

  12. _____

  13. _____

  14. _____

D. Application Exercise

1. Below are several suggested research articles. Read one or more of these articles, paying special attention to the Conclusions/Implications section of the report. Evaluate the extent to which you believe the researchers' discussion would facilitate use of the study findings in clinical settings. If possible, suggest some clinical implications that the researchers did not discuss.

   - Bozoky, I., & Corwin, E. J. (2002). Fatigue as a predictor of postpartum depression. *Journal of Obstetric, Gynecologic, and Neonatal Nursing, 31,* 436–443.
   - Champion, J. D., Shain, R. N., Piper, J., & Perdue, S. T. (2002). Psychological distress among abused minority women with sexually transmitted diseases. *Journal of the American Academy of Nurse Practitioners, 14,* 316–324.
   - Fuller, B. F. (2002). Infant gender differences regarding acute established pain. *Clinical Nursing Research, 11,* 190–203.
   - Perry, J. (2002). Wives giving care to husbands with Alzheimer's disease: A process of interpretive caring. *Research in Nursing & Health, 25,* 307–316.
   - Schultz, A. A., Drew, D., & Hewitt, H. (2002). Comparison of normal saline and heparinized saline for patency of IV locks in neonates. *Applied Nursing Research, 15,* 28–34.
   - Wakefield, B. J. (2002). Risk for acute confusion on hospital admission. *Clinical Nursing Research, 11,* 153–172.

E. Special Projects

1. Select a study from the nursing research literature. Using the criteria indicated in Box 27-2 of the textbook, assess the potential for using the study results in a clinical practice setting. If the study meets the three major classes of criteria for implementation potential, develop a utilization plan.

2. Read the following meta-analytic integrative review:

   Floyd, J. A., Medler, S. M., Ager, J. W., & Janisse, J. J. (2000). Age-related changes in initiation and maintenance of sleep: A meta-analysis. *Research in Nursing & Health, 23,* 106–117.

   Now, search the literature for studies published *after* this meta-analysis. Are the new study results consistent with the conclusions drawn in the integrative review?

3. Search for and evaluate evidence on a topic of your choice.

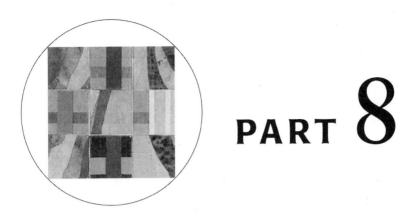

PART 8

Research Reports

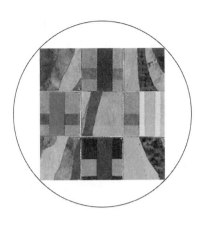

Efficacy and Safety of Sucrose for Procedural Pain Relief in Preterm and Term Neonates

Sharyn Gibbins

Bonnie Stevens

Ellen Hodnett

Janet Pinelli

Arne Ohlsson

Gerarda Darlington

Background: *Preterm and acutely ill term neonates who are hospitalized in a neonatal intensive care unit are subjected to multiple frequent invasive and painful procedures aimed at improving their outcome. Although several trials to determine the efficacy of sucrose for managing procedural pain in preterm and acutely ill term neonates have been developed, these have generally lacked methodological rigor and have not provided clinicians with clear practice guidelines.*

Objectives: *To compare the efficacy and safety of three interventions for relieving procedural pain associated with heel lances in preterm and term neonates, and to explore the influence of contextual factors including sex, severity of illness, and prior painful procedures on pain responses.*

Reprinted with permission from *Nursing Research* (2002;51[6]:375–382).

Methods: *In a randomized controlled trial, 190 neonates were stratified by gestational age and then randomized to receive (a) sucrose and non-nutritive sucking (n = 64), (b) sucrose alone (n = 62), or (c) sterile water and nonnutritive sucking (control) (n = 64) to evaluate the efficacy (pain response as measured using the Premature Infant Pain Profile) (Stevens, Johnson, Petryshen, & Taddio, 1996) and safety (adverse events) following a scheduled heel lance during the first week of life. Stratification was used to control for the effects of age on pain response.*

Results: *Significant differences in pain response existed among treatment groups (F = 22.49, p < .001), with the lowest mean Premature Infant Pain Profile scores in the sucrose and nonnutritive sucking group. Efficacy of sucrose following a heel lance was not affected by severity of illness, postnatal age, or number of painful procedures. Intervention group and sex explained 12% of the variance in Premature Infant Pain Profile scores. Few adverse events occurred (n = 6), and none of them required medical or nursing interventions*

Conclusions: *The combination of sucrose and nonnutritive sucking is the most efficacious intervention for single heel lances. Research on the effects of gestational age on the efficacy and safety of repeated doses of sucrose is required.*

Key Words: *neonates • nonnutritive sucking • pain • sucrose*

Approximately 7–10% of neonates are born preterm (36 weeks gestation or less) and admitted to neonatal intensive care units (NICUs). Many full-term neonates are also hospitalized in NICUs for surgical or medical management of disease processes. Over the past decade, the technological and pharmacological advances in NICUs have increased the survival rates for these high-risk neonates (Philip, 1995). However, the incidence of painful tissue-damaging procedures to improve their survival has also increased. The ability of clinicians to effectively manage pain associated with these procedures has been greatly hindered by lack of high-quality evidence on the safety and efficacy of pain relieving strategies.

PAIN

Pain is defined by the International Association for the Study of Pain (IASP, 1979) as an unpleasant sensory and emotional experience associated with actual or potential tissue damage or described in terms of such damage. A recent "Note" has been added to the IASP definition that states that the inability to communicate in no way negates the possibility that an individual is experiencing pain and is in need of appropriate pain-relieving treatment. Therefore, the issue is no longer that neonates are incapable of pain according to the IASP definition but rather that they must rely on others to make inferences from behavioral and physiological indices for the assessment and management of pain.

The physiological responses to pain involve activation of the sympathetic nervous system (Stevens, 1993; Stevens, Johnston & Horton, 1994). The most common physiological pain responses for preterm and term neonates include: (a) increases in heart rate, respiratory rate, and intracranial pressure; (b) decreases in vagal tone and oxygen saturation; (c) changes in blood pressure; and (d) alterations in autonomic nervous system function (e.g., changes in skin color, nausea, vomiting, palmar sweating, and dilated pupils). These pain indicators have been widely studied in neonates; however, they may be difficult to interpret alone, as they can be influenced by nonpainful stimuli.

Behavioral responses to pain include facial expression, cry, and body movement. However, the quality of behaviors is dependent on gestational age and maturity. Preterm or acutely ill infants may lack sufficient energy to demonstrate body movements in response to pain. Their movements are less organized and less observable than healthy term infants (Craig, Whitfield, Grunau, Linton, & Hadjistavropoulos, 1993; Grunau, Holsti, Whitfield, & Ling, 2000; Johnston & Stevens, 1996). Similarly, cry characteristics may not be an appropriate indicator of pain in preterm or acutely ill neonates who are often unable or too immature to produce a robust cry. However, several studies have demonstrated that irrespective of gestational age, brow bulge, eye squeeze and nasolabial furrow are reliable indicators of pain (Stevens, 1993). Although preterm neonates are less robust than their full-term counterparts, their facial expressions can be used as a valid measure of pain.

Significant hormonal and metabolic responses have been measured in fetuses (Giannakoulopoulos, Sepulveda, Pourtis, Glover, & Fisk, 1994; Teixeira, Fogliani, Giannakoulopoulos, Glover, & Fisk, 1996), and in preterm (Stevens & Johnston, 1994) and term (Anand, Phil, & Hickey, 1992; Kehlet, Brandt, & Rem, 1980; Porter, Wolf, & Miller, 1999) neonates. During painful procedures, these responses stimulate the release of "stress hormones" (e.g., catecholamines, corticosteroids, cortisol, growth hormones, glucagons, epinephrine, and norepinephrine) that increase heart rate and blood pressure, enhance liver and muscle glycogen breakdown, stimulate metabolic rate and improve mental activity (Anand & Hickey, 1987; Anand et al., 1992). Although these biochemical responses have shown an increase in preterm and term neonates in response to pain (Anand et al., 1992; Gunnar, Fisch & Korsvik, 1981), there are limited data on the normal ranges of these hormones, marked variability in the degree of changes between baseline and pain event, and difficulty in measuring these indicators in the clinical setting. In summary, neither physiological, behavioral, or biochemical indicators, when used alone, are valid, reliable, sensitive, or practical for identifying the existence, intensity, location, and impact of pain for a given population or situation (Stevens, 1993). Therefore, pain measurement from a multidimensional perspective appears to be the most appropriate approach.

SUCROSE

The administration of sucrose has been the most frequently studied nonpharmacological intervention for the relief of procedural pain in newborn infants. Sucrose is a sweet disaccharide consisting of fructose and glucose. The calming effect of sucrose is thought to influence endogenous opioid mediation, activated through taste receptors at the tip of the tongue, and nonopioid systems (Blass & Hoffmeyer, 1991). Indirect evidence for endogenous opioid mediation has been derived primarily through studies with animal models (Blass & Shide, 1994; Panksepp, Siviy & Normansell, 1986). Sucrose is altered in the presence of narcotic antagonists, effective with a short latency and effective after the painful stimulus has ceased.

Taste-induced analgesia in animal and human newborns is rapid, enduring, and dependent on the ability to detect sweet taste. Sucrose administered to preterm neonates via a nasogastric tube into the stomach failed to produce analgesia for heel lances compared to an oral route of sucrose administration (Ramenghi, Evans, & Levene, 1999). Sucrose is hydrolyzed into glucose and fructose through the intestinal epithelium that is present by 26 weeks gestation (Naqui, Biskinis, & Khattack, 1999). Given the rapid effects of intraoral sucrose, it is unlikely that hydrolysis in the small intestine is responsible for its pain relieving properties. Taste appears to mediate the opioid response.

Two systematic reviews (Stevens, Taddio, Ohlsson & Einarson, 1997; Stevens & Ohlsson, 1998) have addressed the efficacy of sucrose for procedural pain in neonates. Sucrose, in a wide range of dosages, was found to decrease individual physiologic and behavioral indicators of pain as well as pain assessed using multivariate composite indexes. However, there was inconsistency in the dose of sucrose that was effective, and therefore, an optimal dose to be used in preterm and/or term infants for procedural pain relief could not be identified. Adverse effects were minimal with the use of sucrose, but the dose or administration method providing the smaller risk for less healthy preterm infants and very low-birth-weight infants is not known.

NONNUTRITIVE SUCKING

Nonnutritive sucking (NNS) is the provision of a pacifier or nonlactating nipple into a neonate's mouth to promote sucking behaviors without the provision of breast milk or formula as nutrition (Blass & Hoffmeyer, 1991; Campos, 1994; DiPietro, Cusson, O'Brien & Fox, 1994). Nonnutritive sucking has only recently been rigorously examined as a pain-relieving intervention. The calming effects of NNS have been observed in human and rat neonates, but the mechanisms underlying effectiveness remain unclear. They probably involve stimulation of orotactile and mechano receptors as a pacifier or nonlactating nipple is introduced into the infant's mouth. Unlike the mechanisms of sucrose, the orotactile-induced analgesia associated with NNS does not appear to be mediated through opioid pathways; it is not affected by the administration of narcotic antagonists, and its efficacy is terminated once sucking has ceased. Researchers have found that NNS reduces cry duration and heart rate during painful procedures (Campos, 1994). Although NNS has affected behavioral responses to pain, physiological responses including cortisol response, heart rate, vagal tone, or oxygen saturation (DiPietro et al., 1994) is not affected. Pinelli and Symington, (1998) examined the efficacy of NNS in a systematic review for many neonatal outcomes. Although preterm neonates who were provided with NNS during gavage feedings were discharged from hospital earlier, the review did not reveal any other benefits of NNS.

SUCROSE AND NONNUTRITIVE SUCKING

Researchers have examined the individual and combined effects of sucrose and NNS for pain-relieving interventions in term neonates (Blass & Ciaramitero, 1994; Allen, White & Walburn, 1996) Relative to sterile water, sucrose has been more effective in reducing behavioral pain responses. There is a trend towards lower pain scores with the combination of sucrose and NNS, but further research using larger sample sizes and composite measures of pain is required. One study (Stevens, Johnston, Franck, Petryshen, Jack, et al., 1999) examined the combined efficacy of sucrose and NNS for relieving procedural pain in preterm neonates ($n = 122$). Significant differences in pain responses (measured by PIPP scores [Stevens, Johnston, Petryshen & Taddio, 1996]) between the pacifier with water and control group ($F = 9.00$, $p < .003$), and pacifier with sucrose and control group ($F = 24.09$, $p < .0001$) were found. There was a trend towards lower PIPP scores with the sucrose and NNS group compared to the water and NNS group ($F = 3.62$, $p < .05$). Investigation of the efficacy of these interventions did not include more mature preterm or acutely ill neonates.

Although there is growing evidence that sucrose is effective in reducing pain responses, it is not clear whether the sucrose alone or a synergistic effect of sucrose with NNS is responsible. In addition, there is a paucity of data for preterm or acutely ill term neonates who may not tolerate larger volumes of a solution without side effects (e.g., aspiration, bradycardia, tachycardia, or desaturations). Several studies (Johnston, Stremler, Horton, & Friedman, 1999; Johnston, Stremler, Stevens, & Horton, 1997; Stevens et al., 1999) have found that small doses of sucrose (0.012 –0.12 g) reduce composite pain scores in neonates < 34 weeks of gestation. However, further research on volume and dose-response for a wide range of neonates is justified. The main purpose of this study was to compare the efficacy and safety of 0.5 ml of 24% sucrose with a pacifier (NNS) with sucrose alone or sterile water and NNS for decreasing procedural pain associated with heel lances in preterm and term neonates. Due to the inclusion of preterm and acutely ill term neonates, the dose of sucrose was half the recommended dose from the meta-analysis (Stevens, Taddio, Ohlsson & Einarson, 1997). A secondary objective was to explore the influence of contextual factors including sex, severity of illness, postnatal age, and prior painful procedures on the efficacy of sucrose. These factors have influenced pain responses in previous studies. The Gate Control Theory (GCT) (Melzack & Wall, 1996), existing knowledge of the developing central nervous system (CNS), and data on factors that influence neonates' pain responses were used as explanatory models to examine effective pain management.

Methods

PARTICIPANTS AND SETTING

During a 16-month period in 1998–1999, 661 neonates from one university-affiliated metropolitan Level III NICU were eligible to participate in the study. Eligible neonates were born between 27 and 43 weeks gestation, < 7 days of age, had 5-minute Apgar scores ≥ 7 or cord pH (arterial or venous) ≥ 7.0, and had not undergone surgery. Neonates were excluded from the study if they (a) had a diagnosed major congenital disorder (e.g., neuromuscular disease, spinal cord injury), (b) had received analgesics or sedatives within 12 hours of enrollment, (c) had received paralytic agents (e.g., pancuronium) or (d) had parents who could not speak English. Neonates were not excluded if they required assisted ventilation, supplemental oxygen, or blood pressure support. Eligible neonates were stratified into three gestational age groups: (a) 27–31 $^6/_7$ weeks, (b) 32–35 $^6/_7$ weeks, and (c) 36–43 weeks. Prognostic stratification for gestational age was used only to control for the effects of maturity at birth on the primary outcome, pain. Although other variables may have influenced PIPP scores, sufficient knowledge of neonates' pain responses based on developing neuroanatomy exist, and stratification for gestational age was a biologically plausible variable that may affect pain responses. Four hundred and fifty-two neonates were not recruited for the study (as their particular age stratum was full), parents of seven neonates refused participation (3%), and data for 12 neonates were lost to follow-up (due to equipment failure), leaving 190 neonates in the final sample. Of the 190 neonates enrolled in the study, no differences were found between those neonates who were not recruited, those whose parents refused participation, and those who were lost to follow-up.

The primary outcome of pain response, using the PIPP, was used to calculate the sample size. Using data from one prior study (Stevens et al., 1999), a reduction of 2 points on the PIPP score at 30 seconds following the painful procedure, (approximately 20% on mean observed scores) was considered clinically significant. A sample size of 186 (62 neonates per group) was required.

OUTCOME MEASURES

Efficacy. Efficacy was measured by assessing the infant's pain measured by a validated composite measure, the PIPP (Stevens et al., 1996). The PIPP was specifically developed for preterm neonates and term neonates, and includes the physiological, behavioral, and contextual indicators that have been the most consistent with neonates' pain responses across many research studies (Abu-Saad, Bours, Stevens et al., 1998; Stevens, et al. 1997; Stevens, Johnston, & Gibbins, 2000). The PIPP was derived from multiple data sets and has been shown to have face and content validity and evidence of beginning construct validity for preterm neonate pain measurement of various gestational ages (Ballantyne, Stevens, McAllister, Dionne, & Jack, 1999). In the PIPP, the physiological indicators of pain include the change from baseline in maximum *heart rate* and minimum *oxygen saturation.* The behavioral indicators of pain include the change from baseline in *brow bulge, eye squeeze,* and *naso-labial furrow.* The contextual indicators of pain include *behavioral state* at baseline and *gestational age* at the time of data collection. Indicators in the PIPP are numerically scored on a 4-point composite scale (0, 1, 2, 3) 30 seconds following an acute painful stimulus. Subsequent PIPP scores are obtained every 30 seconds by comparing changes from baseline physiological and behavioral indicators. The number of PIPP scores is dependent on the duration of the painful procedure. The higher the PIPP score, the greater the pain response. For all neonates, a score of < 6 is considered minimal pain and a score > 12 indicates moderate-to-severe pain (the range of scores is 0 to 21). Stevens et al. (1996) discuss instrument development and initial validation in more detail.

Safety. Safety was measured by determining the nature and incidence of adverse events, including: (a) choking, coughing, or vomiting following the administration of sucrose; (b) sustained tachycardia (heart rate > 200) or bradycardia (heart rate < 80) for > 15 seconds following the administration of sucrose; (c) sustained tachypnea (respiratory rate > 80) or dyspnea (respiratory rate < 20) for > 15 seconds following the administration of sucrose; or (d) sustained oxygen desaturation < 80% for > 15 seconds following the administration of sucrose. The safety criteria were attached to each neonate's medical record and any adverse effects were recorded. A safety committee was established prior to study commencement. The members of the safety committee reviewed each adverse event, and rules for stopping the trial included severe choking or need for immediate medical intervention (e.g., intubation or resuscitation).

Severity of Illness. The Score for Neonatal Acute Physiology (SNAP: PE) was used as a measure of severity of neonatal illness. The SNAP: PE is comprised of indicators including birth weight, Apgar score at 5 minutes, and small for gestational age, as well as 26 items based on laboratory tests and vital signs. The SNAP: PE has been validated on over 27,000 infants in 31 NICUs in Canada and the USA (Richardson, Corcoran, Excobar, & Lee, 2000) and has been used in previous studies using the PIPP.

Other Data. Other data such as the neonate's birth weight, sex, gestational age and frequency of prior painful procedures were obtained from the medical records. Data were collected prior to randomization and used to describe the representativeness of the study sample.

PROCEDURE

The efficacy of sucrose and NNS, sucrose alone, and water and NNS were compared in a randomized control trial using a centralized randomization table. Following ethical approval by the combined Research Ethics Board of the university and the university-affiliated institution, parental consent to participate in the study was sought. Once parental consent was obtained, the research pharmacist randomized neonates to one of the three intervention groups. All study solutions were prepared under sterile conditions, labeled as "study drug," and delivered to the neonates' bedside immediately prior to the scheduled heel lance. Based on the literature to support the use of sucrose and/or NNS, it was considered unethical to deny neonates a form of treatment. Therefore, sterile water and the provision of NNS were used for the control group. Because of the study design and intentional lack of a control group (i.e., sterile water alone or no treatment), blinding of the intervention was only possible for the two groups who received a pacifier. To minimize variation, the heel lance procedure was standardized by phases: (a) baseline, (b) intervention, (c) warming, (d) lance, (e) squeeze, and (f) return to baseline. In addition, one individual performed all but five (97%) of the heel lances. The stimulus (heel lance), procedure, and automated lancet were consistent throughout the study period;

however, the use of pacifiers at other times in the NICU was not controlled for due to ethical consideration. The duration of the squeeze phase was dependent on the amount of blood required for the scheduled test, and hence not standardized across groups.

Neonates in the sucrose and NNS group received 0.5 ml of 24% sucrose via a syringe onto the anterior surface of the tongue followed immediately by the insertion of a Wee Soothie pacifier (Children's Medical Ventures, Inc., Weymouth, MA) into the mouth. The pacifier was held in place by the investigator or a research assistant as required 2 minutes before, during, and 5 minutes following the heel lance. The research assistant encouraged sucking by gentle, rhythmic motion of the pacifier, but data on ability to suck efficiently were not collected and may be considered a limitation in the present study. Neonates in the sucrose group received 0.5 ml of 24% sucrose via a syringe onto the anterior surface of the tongue 2 minutes prior to a heel lance. No pacifier was offered. Neonates in the sterile water and NNS group received the identical intervention as neonates randomized to the sucrose and NNS group with the exception of receiving 0.5 ml of sterile water instead of 24% sucrose. Neonates in each intervention group were positioned with their knees flexed towards their chest, arms close to midline and contained in a blanket to prevent large body movements. Only the foot to be used for the heel lance was accessible.

The physiological indicators of pain were recorded by using a SATMASTER™ data collection system ("EMG," Los Angeles, CA) that provides descriptive statistics for each phase of the heel lance procedure. Data were recorded by the SATMASTER™ system second-to-second and transmitted into a personal computer. The behavioral indicators of pain were recorded on videotape with a zoom lens (Sony digital zoom, handycam vision, 72X). Prior to the scheduled heel lance, the neonate's behavioral state, baseline heart rate, and oxygen saturation were recorded. An oxygen saturation monitor (Pulse Oximeter, Model N-3000, Hayward, CA) was applied to the neonate's hand or foot to record the heart rate and oxygen saturation. For each data collection session, the investigator calibrated the neonate's ECG monitor with the pulse oximeter and the SATMASTER™ system. If there was a discrepancy in the recorded heart rates (> 10 beats/minute) between the monitors (detected by the research assistant at the time of data collection), the data were collected manually by the research assistant using a preprinted and standardized form with 5-second time increments. Having the data collector enter a marker into the SATMASTER™ program simultaneously with a verbal command onto the videotape synchronized physiological and behavioral indicators.

Behavioral facial data were videotaped in real time, copied, and forwarded to a facial coder who had been specially trained in facial coding and who was kept uninformed to the purpose of the study, phases of the heel lance procedure, and group allocation (in the case of the two pacifier groups). An experienced coder did regular intra-rater reliability and validity checks after approximately 25 neonates were randomized. The intra-rater reliability was high (alpha = 0.93). The research assistant who performed the heel lance procedure and collected data from the neonate's medical record did not know which solution the neonate was receiving with a pacifier.

The PIPP scores were manually computed from the raw physiological SATMAS-TER™ data and facial coding. The calculation of all PIPP scores were double-checked by two research assistants and double entered into a data management system by two separate research assistants blinded to group allocation. All data were verified for completeness. Logic checks were performed on the individual databases and there was a very low error rate in data entry (less than 1%). Manual calculation of physiological data (for discrepancies in heart rate between monitors) was required for eight neonates.

Results

Data were analyzed using the SPSS™ statistical package (Norusis, 1993). Representativeness of the sample was first determined by comparing data from the eligible refusers to those neonates who participated in the study. Later, comparing the study sample to the annual statistics from the study hospital's 1999 perinatal database determined representativeness of the sample. Neonates who were lost to follow up due to equipment failure recognized at the time of facial coding were compared to study participants and no differences were found. Demographic and other baseline variables were compared between treatment groups and descriptive statistics were calculated. There were no differences in any of the baseline variables. Data were then subjected to a repeated measures analysis of variance (RM ANOVA), using the PIPP scores, to determine the efficacy of the treatment groups over time. The significance level for all tests was set at 0.05. To explore the influence of contextual factors on pain response, a hierarchical regression analysis was performed (Table 1).

RESULTS BY RESEARCH QUESTION

The Most Efficacious Method of Sucrose Delivery for Neonates Experiencing a Heel Lance. All neonates had a PIPP score at 30 seconds and 96% had PIPP scores at 60 seconds. Subsequent PIPP scores were not available because only 60% of the

Table 1   *Description of Sample Characteristics by Intervention Group*

Characteristic	Sucrose & NNS (*n* = 64)	Sucrose (*n* = 62)	Water & NNS (*n* = 64)
GA (weeks)	33.69 (3.84)	33.9 (3.83)	33.67 (4.05)
Weight (g)	2207 (924)	2286 (1002)	2242 (943)
Age at enrollment (days)	3.12 (1.85)	3.02 (1.75)	2.67 (1.89)
SNAP: PE	4.14 (4.56)	4.68 (6.73)	4.00 (5.02)
Number of painful procedures	11.86 (2.21)	11.63 (2.3)	11.92 (1.56)
Duration of procedure (min)	11.13 (1.68)	10.68 (1.21)	10.92 (1.26)
Number of males	30 (47%)	32 (51%)	32 (50%)

Note. All values are expressed as means (*SD*) or percentages as indicated. NNS = nonnutritive sucking; GA = gestational age; SNAP: PE = severity of illness.

data were available at 90 seconds and 40% of the data were available at 120 seconds (as the duration of procedure varied). The results are summarized in Table 2. A RM ANOVA was performed to determine the efficacy of the three interventions for reducing procedural pain. The pain scores (PIPP) at 30 and 60 seconds were used as the dependent variable. The between-subject factor was the intervention group and the within-subjects factor was time. There was a significant main effect of intervention group ($F = 22.49$, $p < .001$). There was no main effect of time and no interaction between treatment intervention and time ($F = 1.69$, $p < .12$). Post hoc analyses were performed to contrast the treatment interventions with each other. The PIPP scores were significantly lower in the sucrose and NNS compared to sucrose alone ($p < .002$) or sterile water and NNS ($p < .001$). No significant differences in PIPP scores between sucrose alone or sterile water and NNS groups were found ($p = .57$).

Determining the Nature and Incidence of Adverse Effects by Treatment Group. Due to the small number of adverse events ($n = 6$), only frequencies and percentages of adverse events by phase were calculated. Three neonates in the sucrose alone group desaturated during the study period, two neonates in the water and NNS group desaturated during the study period, and one neonate choked on the pacifier. No adverse events occurred with neonates randomized to the sucrose and NNS group. More adverse events occurred in the least mature neonates ($n = 4$) compared to the middle ($n = 1$) and most mature ($n = 1$) neonates.

Factors That Influence Pain Responses. A hierarchical multiple regression analysis was used to determine which variables contributed to the variance in the major outcome pain, as assessed by 30 second PIPP scores. Variables were entered sequentially into the model depending on the potential contribution to the variance in PIPP scores. The intervention group was entered first as contributing potential to the variance in PIPP scores. Neonatal characteristics that have been shown to influence pain response in previous studies (e.g., the number of painful procedures, post natal age, severity of illness, and sex) were entered last. Gestational age and behavioral state were not entered into the model, as they were contextual indicators used to compute the PIPP score. The intervention group explained 9% of the variance and sex explained 3% of the variance. All other variables were deleted from the final model, as they did not add

Table 2 *Composite Pain Responses at 30 and 60 Seconds by Intervention Group*

	Mean (*SD*) PIPP score	
Intervention Group	**30 seconds**	**60 seconds**
Sucrose and NNS	8.16 (3.24) (*n* = 64)	8.78 (4.03) (*n* = 60)
Sucrose alone	9.77 (3.04) (*n* = 62)	11.20 (3.25) (*n* = 57)
Sterile water and NNS	10.19 (2.67) (*n* = 64)	11.20 (3.47) (*n* = 59)

Note. All values expressed as means (standard deviation); PIPP = Premature Infant Pain Profile; NNS = nonnutritive sucking.

information in the presence of sex and intervention group. There were associations between sex and PIPP scores, with male neonates scoring significantly higher PIPP scores than female neonates. The mean PIPP score for males was 9.73 (2.92) and 9.01 (3.25) for females; however, the differences were small and not clinically significant.

Discussion

Although pain management for neonates has improved over the last few decades, many painful procedures such as heel lance continue to be performed on neonates without appropriate analgesia or comfort measures. The suboptimal management of pain is related to misconceptions and myths of neonates' capacity to detect, transmit, and interpret pain as well as concerns about safety of analgesics. Administration of analgesics to neonates requires careful consideration of the pharmacokinetics (movement of drugs in the body over time) and pharmacodynamics (dose-response relationship) of the specific agent (Stevens, Johnson & Franck, 2000). In addition, developmental differences between the metabolic functions of preterm and term neonates' must be considered prior to the administration of analgesics. All neonates in this study received a form of pain management for heel lances. Heel lances were chosen because they are the most commonly performed painful procedure in the NICU. Sucrose was hypothesized to reduce pain by opioid mediation, activated by taste. The NNS was hypothesized to reduce pain by tactile mechanisms, while the combination of sucrose and NNS was hypothesized to offer the most efficacious pain relief.

Sucrose and NNS significantly reduced PIPP scores for heel lances in preterm and term neonates at 30 seconds. These results are generally consistent with comparative studies where differences in pain responses between term (Abad, Diaz, Domenech, Robayna, Rico et al., 1993; Haouari, Wood, Griffiths & Levene, 1995) and preterm (Johnston et al., 1999; Stevens et al., 1999) neonates who received sucrose or water for pain associated with heel lances have been observed. The PIPP scores were also lowest in the sucrose and NNS group at 60 seconds; however, they generally increased from scores obtained at 30 seconds. As procedures become more invasive, as measured by duration of procedure and/or intensity of pain, the magnitude of physiological and behavioral responses increase. Porter et al. (1999) also reported that the magnitude of physiological and behavioral change is not affected by gestational age; neonates of all gestational ages can differentiate procedural invasiveness. Similarly, neonates of all gestational ages can demonstrate increased magnitude in response to increased duration (in seconds to minutes) of the procedure. These results are consistent with the present study. Although the present study did not have sufficient power to examine the influence of gestational age on the efficacy of sucrose, neonates in each gestational age stratum indicated a trend towards higher PIPP scores at 60 seconds, suggesting that the prolonged squeeze phase is more invasive than the lance phase. Further research comparing PIPP scores by gestational age over a longer duration of time is required.

A joint statement of the Fetus and Newborn Committee, Canadian Paediatric Society and the American Academy of Pediatrics has provided guidelines for pharmacological pain management in neonates. The administration of sucrose and pacifier are recommended approaches to pain relief for heel lances in preterm and term neonates. Sucrose and NNS are readily available in hospital nurseries, inexpensive, easily administered, and safe. In addition, the long history of use of sweet solutions and pacifiers for painful procedures further increase the likelihood of acceptance of sucrose and NNS as routine interventions for pain management in the NICU. Given the rapid and enduring effects of sucrose and NNS, they can be given together in advance of minor to moderate procedural pain. Although sucrose and NNS is not efficacious for moderate-to-severe pain, the combined therapy can be used as an adjunct with pharmacological interventions.

Other factors that have been shown to influence pain responses, such age at study session, severity of illness, or previous painful procedures were included in the present study; however, they did not appear to modulate pain responses. Sex explained some of the variance in PIPP scores, with male neonates having statistically but not clinically significant higher pain scores.

In summary, three treatment interventions were compared for the management of procedural pain in preterm and term neonates. The most efficacious and safe intervention was 0.5 ml 24% sucrose and NNS. Although there were a few adverse events during the study period, they were benign in nature, resolved spontaneously, and did not require medical or nursing intervention. In light of the relatively simple, yet efficacious, intervention to manage neonatal pain, changes in pain practice for selective painful procedures could easily be incorporated into standard NICU care. However, research on additional interventions that could be used in combination with sucrose and NNS is required in order to better reduce the pain associated with heel lances. In addition, the efficacy and safety of repeated doses of sucrose and NNS (alone or in combination with other interventions) for a variety of painful procedures is needed. Research is also needed on the management of pain for other high-risk neonates, such as preterm neonates less than 27 weeks gestation, cognitively impaired, or those with existing disease processes.

Accepted for publication May 23, 2002.

The authors thank the Hospital for Sick Children, Toronto Ontario, Canada for the Research Training Award (Sharyn Gibbins, PhD, Sunnybrook & Women's College Health Sciences Centre, Toronto, Ontario, Canada) and the Ontario Ministry of Health, Toronto, Ontario, Canada for the Career Scientist Award (Bonnie Stevens, PhD, Hospital for Sick Children, Toronto, Ontario, Canada), and the staff and families at Sunnybrook & Women's College Health Sciences Centre, Toronto, Ontario, Canada.

Corresponding author: Sharyn Gibbins, RN, PhD, Sunnybrook & Women's College Health Sciences Centre, 76 Grenville Street, Room 445, Toronto, Ontario, Canada M5A 1B2.

References

Abad. F., Diaz, N. M., Domenech, E., Robayna, M., Rico, J., Arrecivita, A. et al. (1993). *Attenuation of pain-related behavior in neonates given oral sweet solutions*. 7th World Congress on Pain, Paris (Abstract).

Abu-Saad, H., Bours, G., Stevens, B. et al. (1998). Assessment of pain in the neonate. *Semin Perinatol, 22*, 402-416.

Allen, K., White, D., & Walburn, J. (1996). Sucrose as an analgesic agent for infants during immunization injections. *Archives of Pediatrics and Adolescent Medicine, 150*, 270-274.

Anand, K., & Hickey, P. R. (1987). Randomized trial of high-dose sufentanil aesthesia in neonates undergoing cardiac surgery: Effects on the metabolic stress response. *Anesthesiology, 67*, 502A.

Anand, K., Phil, D., & Hickey, P.R. (1992). Halothane-morphine compared with high-dose sufentanil for anesthesia and postoperative analgesia in neonatal cardiac surgery. *New England Journal of Medicine, 326*, 1-9.

Ballantyne, M., Stevens, B., McAllister, M., Dionne, D., & Jack, A. (1999). Validation of the premature infant pain profile in the clinical setting. *The Clinical Journal of Pain, 15*, 297-303.

Blass, E., & Ciaramitaro, V. (1994). A new look at some old mechanisms in human newborns: Taste and tactile determinants of state, affect and action. *Monographs of the Society for Research in Child Development, 59*, 1-80.

Blass, E. & Hoffmeyer, L. B. (1991). Sucrose as an analgesic for newborn infants. *Pediatrics, 87(2)*, 215-220.

Campos, R. (1994) Rocking and pacifiers: Two comforting interventions for heelstick pain.*Research in Nursing and Health, 17(1)*, 321-331.

Craig, K. Whitfield, M. F., Grunau, R. V., Linton, J., & Hadjistavropoulos, H. (1993). Pain in the preterm neonate: behavioral and physiological indices. *Pain, 52*, 287-299.

DiPietro, J. A., Cusson, R. M., O'Brien, M., & Fox, N. A. (1994). Behavioral and physiologic effects of nonnutritive sucking during gavage feeding in preterm infants. *Pediatric Research, 36(2)*, 207-214.

Giannakoulopoulos, X., Sepulveda, W., Pourtis, P., Glover, V., & Fisk, N. M. (1994). Fetal plasma cortisol and B-endorphin response to intrauterine needling. *Lancet, 344*, 77-80.

Gibbins, S. & Stevens, B. (2001). Mechanisms of sucrose and nonnutritive sucking in procedural pain management in infants. *Pain Research & Management. 6(1)*, 21-28.

Grunau, R., Holsti, L., Whitfield, M., & Ling, E. (2000). Are twitches, startles and body movements pain indicators in expremely low birth weight infants? *Clinical Journal of Pain, 16(1)*, 37-45.

Gunnar, M., Fisch, R., & Korsvik, S. (1981). The effects of circumcision on serum cortisol and behavior. *Psychoneuroendocrinology, 6*, 269-275.

Haouari, N., Wood, C., Griffiths, G., & Levene, M. (1995). The analgesic effect of sucrose in full term infants: A randomized controlled trial. *British Medical Journal, 310*, 1498-1500.

Johnston, C. & Stevens, B. (1996). Experience in a neonatal intensive care unit affects pain response. *Pediatrics, 98*(5), 925-930.

Johnston, C., Stremler, R .L., Horton, L. J., & Friedman, A. (1999). Effect of repeated doses of sucrose during heel stick procedure in preterm neonates. *Biology of the Neonate, 75,* 160-166.

Johnston, C., Stremler, R. L., Stevens, B. J. & Horton, L. J. (1997). Effectiveness of oral sucrose and simulated rocking on pain response in preterm neonates. *Pain, 72*(1), 193-199.

Kehlet, H., Brandt, M. & Rem, J. (1980). Role of neurogenic stimuli in mediating the endocrine-metabolic response to surgery. *Journal of Parenteral and Enteral Nutrition, 4,* 152-156.

Melzack, R., & Wall, P. (1996). Pain mechanisms: A new theory. A gate control system modulates sensory input from the skin before it evokes pain perception and response... reprinted with permission from *Science 150:*971-979, 1965. *Pain Forum, 5*(1), 3-11.

Naqui, M., Biskinis, E. & Khattack, I. (1999). Effects of 50% sucrose on pain responses in full-term male infants during circumcision. *Pediatric Academic Societies' annual meeting* (abstract) Norusis, N. (1993). *SPSS for Windows: Base System User's Guide.* Release 6.0. Chicago: SPSS Inc.

Panksepp, J., Siviy, S. & Normansell, L. (1986). Brain opioids and social emotion. In M. Reite and T. Fields (Eds.), *The psychobiology of attachment and separation* (pp.3-39). San Diego, CA. Academic Press.

Pinelli, J. & Symington, A. (1998) Non nutritive sucking in premature infants. In J. C. Sinclair, M. B. Bracken, R. S. Soll, J. D. Horbar (Eds.). *Neonatal Modules of the Cochrane Data Base of Systematic Reviews.* (Updated February, 1998). Available in the Cochrane Library (Data base on disk and CD ROM). The Cochrane Collaboration; Issue 4, Oxford: Update Software; 1998. Updated quarterly.

Philip, A. G. S. (1995). Neonatal mortality rate: Is further improvement possible? *Journal of Pediatrics, 126,* 427-433.

Porter, F., Wolf, C., & Miller, P. (1999). Procedural pain in newborn infants: the influence of intensity and development. *Pediatrics, 104*(1), 313-19.

Ramenghi, E., & Levene, M (1999). Sucrose analgesia: Absorptive mechanism or taste perception? *Arch Dis Child Fetal Neonatal Ed, 80,* F146-F147.

Richardson, D., Corcoran, J., Escobar, G. & Lee, S. (2000). SNAP-II & SNAP: PE-newborn illness severity and mortality risk scores. *Journal of Pediatrics, 137,* 617-624.

Stevens, B. (1993). *Physiological and behavioral responses of premature infants to a tissue-damaging stimulus.* Unpublished doctoral dissertation, Montreal: McGill University.

Stevens, B., & Johnston, C. (1994). Physiological responses of preterm infants to a painful stimulus *Nursing Research, 43,* 226-231.

Stevens, B., Johnston, C., & Franck, L. (2000). *The use of sucrose and pacifiers for managing neonatal pain: Are we alleviating pain or conditioning the infant.* Abstract #5. ISPP2000, the 5th international symposium on paediatric pain. London, UK.

Stevens, B., Johnston, C., & Gibbins, S. (2000). Pain assessment in neonates. In K. J. S.Anand, B. J.Stevens and P. J. McGrath (Eds), *Pain in neonates 2nd* revised and enlarged edition (pp. 101-135). Amsterdam: Elsevier Science B.V.

Stevens, B., Johnston, C. C., & Horton, L. (1994). Factors that influence the behavioral pain responses of premature infants. *Pain, 59*, 101-109.

Stevens, B., Johnston, C., Franck, L., Petryshen, P., Jack, A., & Foster, G. (1999). The efficacy of developmentally sensitive interventions and sucrose for relieving procedural pain in very low birth weight neonates. *Nursing Research 48*(1), 35-42.

Stevens, B., Johnston, C. C., Petryshen, P., & Taddio, A. (1996). Premature infant pain profile: development and initial validation. *Clinical Journal of Pain, 12,* 13-22.

Stevens, B., & Ohlsson, A. (1998). The efficacy of sucrose to reduce procedural pain in neonates as assessed by physiologic and/or behavioral outcomes. In J. C. Sinclair, M. B. Bracken, R. S. Soll, J. D. Horbar (Eds.). *Neonatal Modules of the Cochrane Data Base of Systematic Reviews.* (Updated February, 1998). Available in the Cochrane Library (Data base on disk and CD ROM). The Cochrane Collaboration; Issue 2, Oxford: Update Software; 1998. Updated quarterly.

Stevens, B., Taddio, A., Ohlsson, A. & Einarson, T. (1997). The efficacy of sucrose for relieving procedural pain in neonates: A systematic review and meta-analysis. *Acta Paediatrica, 86,* 837-842.

Teixeira, J., Fogliani, R., Giannakoulopoulos, X., Glover, V., & Fisk, N. (1996). Fetal haemodynamic stress response to invasive procedures. *Lancet, 347,* 624.

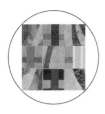

Carrying On

The Experience of Premature Menopause in Women With Early Stage Breast Cancer

M. Tish Knobf

Background: *The survival benefit of adjuvant chemotherapy for breast cancer is established but the experience of organ system toxicity for women, specifically ovarian toxicity, is not fully known.*

Objectives: *The purpose of the study was to develop a substantive theory that would describe and explain women's responses to chemotherapy-induced premature menopause within the context of breast cancer.*

Methods: *Qualitative inquiry with Grounded Theory methodology was used to collect, code, and analyze the data. The purposive sample consisted of 27 women with early stage breast cancer who received adjuvant chemotherapy. The majority of women were married, well educated, and employed with a mean age of 41 years. Amenorrhea was reported by 24 women, a peri-menopausal pattern of bleeding was described by two women, and one woman had return of normal menses. Women participated in interviews ranging from 45 minutes to 2 hours and other data sources, such as informal discussions with oncology care providers, and lay women's writings about menopause and midlife women's health were used to increase interpretation of the data.*

Results: *Vulnerability was identified as the basic social psychological problem for women. Carrying On is the basic process that explains how women respond to vulnerability as they attempt to assimilate drug-induced premature menopause into their breast cancer experience. The stages of Carrying On (Being Focused, Facing Uncertainty, Becoming*

Reprinted with permission from *Nursing Research* (2002;51[1]:9–17).

Menopausal, and Balancing) progressed from minimizing the early menopause experience to developing an awareness to balancing the dynamic relationship of menopause and cancer in their lives.
Conclusions: *This study described the complexity of the experience of chemotherapy-induced premature menopause in women with early stage breast cancer and identified gaps in knowledge about menopausal symptom distress and factors influencing symptom management and outcomes in this population. Future research is needed to evaluate interventions during and after adjuvant therapy to improve the quality of survival of women who experience ovarian toxicity related to early stage breast cancer treatment.*
Key Words: *adjuvant therapy • · breast cancer • menopause*

Breast cancer is a significant health problem for midlife women, with an estimated 193,700 cases to be diagnosed in the United States in 2001 (Greenlee, Hill-Harmon, Murray, & Thun, 2001). Postoperative adjuvant chemotherapy has significantly contributed to improved survival in younger women (Early Breast Cancer Trialists Group, 1998), but it is also associated with acute and long-term side effects (Knobf, 1990). Chemotherapy is toxic to the gonads, resulting in menstrual irregularities, amenorrhea and menopausal symptoms (Knobf, 1998; Lin, Aiken, & Good, 1999). Women with breast cancer therapy who experience chemotherapy induced premature menopause report more physical symptom distress and poorer sexual functioning than other breast cancer survivors (Ganz, Rowland, Desmond, Meyerowitz & Watts, 1998; Young-McGaughan, 1996). And, persistent physical complaints are associated with an increased risk of moderate to severe psychological distress in these women (Schag, et al, 1993).

Menopausal symptoms have been identified as part of the symptom profile of women treated with adjuvant therapy for breast cancer, but a full symptom experience has not been described (Larson, et al., 1994). Furthermore, it is important to note that the menopausal transition of midlife women is not merely a symptom experience, but rather a complex, dynamic, biosocial and biophysical phenomenon which is influenced by many factors over time (Voda & George, 1986). This broader perspective of menopause goes beyond symptom distress and recognizes how the context of women's lives shapes the totality of the experience. How young midlife women respond to drug induced premature menopause in the context of newly diagnosed early stage breast cancer and adjuvant chemotherapy is unknown. The purpose of this study was to develop a substantive theory that would describe and explain women's responses to chemotherapy induced premature menopause within the context of breast cancer.

Method

Naturalistic inquiry using grounded theory (GT) methodology was chosen because little is known about the phenomenon (Lincoln & Guba, 1985), context is important in understanding the problem (Munhull & Boyd, 1993) and the axioms posed are consistent with women centered thought and nursing epistemologies (Munhull, 1989; Seibold, Richards, & Simon, 1994; Streubert & Carpenter, 1995; Stern, Allen & Moxley, 1984). Grounded theory method is designed to discover dominant processes that can predict and explain relevant behavior in terms of meaning (Glaser & Strauss, 1967). Meanings arise out of social interactions and grounded theorists search for social psychological processes present in human interactions in order to understand behavior in complex situations (Chenitz & Swanson, 1986; Hutchinson, 1993). The aim of using GT method in this study was to discover the basic social psychological problem for women with breast cancer treatment induced menopause and the social psychological processes used to resolve the problem.

Participants

Following approval of the study by the Institutional Review Board, a potential list of participants who met the inclusion criteria for the initial purposive sample were identified by area oncologists. Women were sent a letter describing the study and inviting them to participate which was followed by a telephone call. Women were selectively sampled based on the following criteria: primary breast cancer diagnosis, adjuvant chemotherapy with or without endocrine therapy (Tamoxifen), premenopausal status at the beginning of adjuvant therapy (defined as menstrual period within the past three months), and documented menstrual irregularities or subjective menopausal symptoms following therapy. The rationale for the initial purposive sample was to examine the phenomenon where it was found to exist, gather data from knowledgeable participants and to obtain data that will capture a wide range of variation (Chenitz & Swanson, 1986; Coyne, 1997). The sample was also restricted to White women because of the effect of culture on the meaning of menopause and interpretation of symptoms (Weber, 1994), Sampling for variation in race, class or gender in qualitative studies should be done only when those variables are deemed analytically important (Glaser, 1978; Sandelowski, 1995).

Based on the analysis of data from the first ten participants, theoretical sampling was then employed to maximize variations in the data, discover the entire range of the phenomenon with confirming and disconfirming cases and to verify relationships among the data (Glaser, 1978). The final sample of participants consisted of 27 women with breast cancer, the majority of whom were married, well educated, and employed with an average age of 40.8 years ($\pm$ 3.7). All women had received chemotherapy, and nine (37%) had endocrine therapy (Tamoxifen) prescribed for five years following chemotherapy. Amenorrhea was reported by 24 women, two women described a perimenopausal pattern of irregular menstrual cycles and one participant experienced amenorrhea with a return of menses a few months after therapy was completed. The average time since the diagnosis of breast cancer was 4.5 years ($\pm$ 0.43) with a range of one to nine years.

Data Collection

Data were collected over a two-year period (3/96 to 3/98) and included participant interviews, informal discussions with specialty physicians and nurses, field notes from national menopause conferences and breast cancer seminars, lay women's writings, and memos. Potential participants were contacted by telephone, the study was further described and a mutually agreed upon location and date were determined for the interview. Following written informed consent, the participants were asked what it was like to experience premature menopause during and after adjuvant chemotherapy for breast cancer. Seven women from the initial purposive sample were contacted a second time to clarify, explore or expand on data generated in the original interview and the remaining 20 women participated in a single interview. Interviews ranged from 45 minutes to 2 hours. All interviews were tape recorded, transcribed verbatim and reviewed for omissions or errors and to make notes on verbal intonations or nonverbal behaviors during the interview.

Data Analysis

The constant comparative method of Grounded Theory was used to simultaneously collect, code and analyze the data (Glaser, 1978; Glaser & Strauss, 1967; Strauss & Corbin, 1990). Three levels of coding were used (Hutchinson, 1993). Analysis of data began with open coding (Glaser, 1978), generating Level I or "in vivo" codes. Level II coding clustered codes by similarities and differences, compared codes across the data set and abstracted phenomena observed, which were labeled as categories. Most of the categories were identified in the analysis of data from the first five to ten interviews, but questioning continued throughout the process with theoretical sampling to densify and saturate the categories (Chentiz & Swanson, 1986; Glaser 1978). Theoretical coding was used to examine the relationships among the categories, aided by schemes and diagrams to see how the categories fit (Glaser, 1978; Strauss & Corbin, 1990). The analytic process of open to theoretical coding is illustrated with selected data from the audit trail from the theoretical construct, Facing Uncertainty, in Figure 1. Selective coding (Level III) focused on the core variable, further establishing the linkages between categories and moving the data to a more abstract level to explain the basic social problem and process (Glaser, 1990).

   Credibility, transferability, dependability and confirmability are four factors necessary to establish trustworthiness of the data (Lincoln & Guba, 1985). These factors were addressed by the following activities: (a) using a senior qualitative researcher who read the initial ten interviews for analytic competence in early level coding and continued as a mentor throughout analytic process; (b) experiential learning for new intellectual skills as a novice qualitative researcher through regular meetings with faculty and graduate students engaged in grounded theory analysis (Benoliel, 1996); (c) using multiple data sources to enhance interpretation of interview data; (d) sharing data with two nonparticipant women from the target population for common findings; (e) developing an audit trail of memos and field

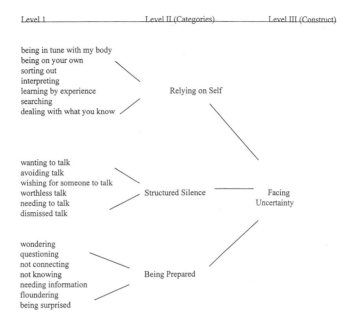

Level 1   Level II (Categories)   Level III (Construct)

being in tune with my body
being on your own
sorting out
interpreting
learning by experience   Relying on Self
searching
dealing with what you know

wanting to talk
avoiding talk
wishing for someone to talk
worthless talk   Structured Silence   Facing
needing to talk   Uncertainty
dismissed talk

FIGURE 1. Selected
code data from audit   wondering
trail for theoretical   questioning
                              not connecting
construct: facing   not knowing   Being Prepared
uncertainty.   needing information
                              floundering
                              being surprised

notes (Rodgers & Cowles, 1993); and (f) using a grounded theory researcher as a
consultant in refining the final theory.

Results

Vulnerability was identified as the basic social psychological problem for women
who experience premature menopause as a consequence of adjuvant treatment.
Vulnerability related to existential concerns from a cancer diagnosis, physical and
psychological responses to chemotherapy side effects, alterations in self concept,
threatened sense of control over one's body and health, uncertainty, unpredictabili-
ty of symptoms and unknown risks of future health problems related to early
menopause. The uncertainty and lack of control of what is happening now and what
might happen in the future are captured in the words of two women: "I think now,
what has happened to my body because of chemotherapy? That is what you have
to live with," and "As time goes on, you think about osteoporosis and heart disease."

The basic social psychological process of premature cancer therapy induced
menopause is Carrying On, which explains how women respond to vulnerability as
they begin to assimilate early menopause into their recovery process from breast
cancer. Four stages were discovered in the process of Carrying On: Being Focused,
Facing Uncertainty, Becoming Menopausal, and Balancing. Each stage is a Level III
code, a theoretical construct that conceptualizes the relationship among all three

level of codes (Hutchinson, 1993). Women did not move through the stages in a distinct linear fashion, but often moved back and forth between stages (Figure 2).

Being Focused

The stage of Being Focused represents the time during chemotherapy treatment. Women are immersed in learning new terms, treatment schedules, new providers and side effects of therapy as they try to maintain normal activities at work and at home. Getting through treatment was the main priority and women repeatedly stated that you do what you have to do, "The focus was really on treatment, raising the children, doing what I had to do." The strategies used by women related to induced menopause at this time were minimizing menopausal symptoms and isolating the meaning of menopause.

Minimizing Menopausal Symptoms. The menopausal symptoms during this stage were secondary to everything else and women tried to ignore them or "do in spite of" them so that they could cope with other issues. "I didn't enjoy the hot flashes, I accepted immediately that I couldn't be helped with hormonal therapy, that was not an option...my attitude was always that this is doable, we can cope with this and do this."

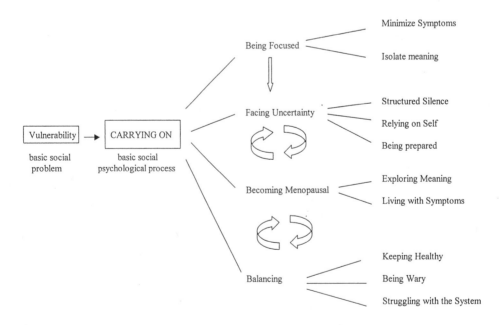

FIGURE 2. Carrying on: a substantive theory about the experience of premature menopause in women with early stage breast cancer.

Isolating Meaning of Menopause. During therapy, women dealt with the onset of menopause objectively, placing any meaning of the event secondary to their cancer experience.

> It (menopause) is secondary when you are going through everything else. You are dealing with a life threatening illness and that is all you can focus on. Then you are getting poisoned. I'm not getting my period; who even notices. So I really think that it is secondary.

> At the time (during chemotherapy), menopause just meant a stop of periods.

Facing Uncertainty

There is a linear relationship between Stage I (Being Focused) and Stage II, which gradually transitions women from the crisis response of doing to "just get through it" to the process and reflection of the actual experience. Some women moved through Stage II while still on therapy while others moved through it sequentially or continuously for months or years following therapy. Uncertainty was the result of women's inability to distinguish what part of the experience was attributable to breast cancer or to menopause and the perception of not knowing and not being able to connect symptoms with meaning or cause. The three conditions in this stage, Structured Silence, Relying on Self and Being Prepared are integrally linked. Uncertainty is inherent in the cancer experience but was intensified for these women because of the menopause. The degree of their uncertainty was related to whether or not they received information about menopause, the inability of providers to predict the symptom experience for an individual woman and the lack of talking about the menopausal experience.

> It is hard to sort out what is what. Is it because you are suddenly deprived of estrogen or is it because you have cancer and you are dealing with a life threatening disease? At first you think it is the cancer, then you think, gee, this could be part of the menopause. But people don't tell you that. They are saying: you are going for treatment, you will be okay..smile..think positive. It is all woven together.

Structured Silence. Physicians informed women of potential alterations in menstrual function at the beginning of chemotherapy, but dialogue about menopause related symptoms thereafter was uncommon. Nurses focused their teaching on the most predictable, high-risk side effects of treatment but did not discuss menopause, unless a woman raised questions. Visits to the oncologist were often characterized by anxiety and a strong focus on the disease and treatment. Standard physician initiated questions dominated many of the interactions.

> Every chemo treatment I was asked, how are you doing? Oh, I guess I am fine. You don't know what is normal and what is abnormal. If they (nurses and physicians) had been more probing in their questions, like are you sleeping at night? Well, no I am not. What's happening when you wake up? Well, I am waking up soaking wet. I'm not waking up to go to the bathroom. A nurse could have pulled that information out of me and recognized this. Hey, wait a minute, this woman is going through

menopause. I shouldn't be home saying, oh my God, I am losing my mind. I'm more bothered by being beet red and sweating than I am from throwing up or being nauseous. They could have pulled out that this was more of an issue for me...they could have helped me through it a lot more.

Women who were symptomatic and sought assistance in managing menopausal symptoms were more upset by the lack of talking and lack of definitive information from oncologists. Some women felt a lack of sensitivity by physicians to listen to their concerns, as one woman describes:

They (physicians) dismiss you because, well it's almost like, why are you worried about this...they don't want to hear any of it..they want to make it a nonissue. They dismiss you like you are a dummy worrying about stupid stuff. They almost make themselves unapproachable about issues like this.

Discussions of menopause with friends or family members also were limited, especially among younger patients who had no peers entering menopause. Some women reported very supportive and validating conversations with other breast cancer patients, usually within the environment of a support group. In general, however, menopause was not openly discussed. "People don't talk about that (menopause). People talk about having babies and what that's like. Now a lot of people talk about breast cancer and chemotherapy. They talk about hot flashes, but they don't talk about other symptoms."

Relying on Self. Women had to rely on their own experience to define and interpret symptoms and hormonal changes. The uncertainty and unpredictable nature of the experience was accentuated by the lack of the oncology specialist's knowledge about menopause.

I found that every time I asked a question, the answer was, well, everybody is different. I never got a clear cut answer. With the diagnosis it was: this is what you have, this is what we are going to do—that was easy. But from there on, it got to be-well-you are on your own here. This is what we are going to do to you but we don't know how your body will react.

Being Prepared. The level of preparation for experiencing induced menopause ranged from not being prepared at all to some degree of preparation. Physicians generally did not describe the various patterns of menstrual irregularities and rarely discussed menopausal symptoms other than hot flashes. For women who were symptomatic, not being well prepared was associated with more emotional distress (Knobf, 1999), but even asymptomatic women would have liked being better prepared for the experience.

I think the element of surprise is partly what you are not prepared for and saying that your periods may stop doesn't sound like you are going to have menopause. It is not the same statement and if doctors are saying that your periods will stop, then they are not giving the full message.

Women expressed a desire to talk about menopause and several women identified nurses as the healthcare professional best suited to provide information and discuss the experience.

I think nurses are probably more responsible in dealing with patients than the doctors on this (menopause). I think that it is the nursing staff who are more probing in their questions. You have to be a little bit more in depth because women are not going to be as open or up front about this.

Becoming Menopausal

In Stage III, women began to explore what menopause meant to them beyond the physiologic event of amenorrhea. Developing awareness of menopause occurred earlier for symptomatic women, as their experience was being defined by symptoms other than menstrual cycle changes. Women moved back and forth between Stages II and III as the menopausal symptom experience was closely related to level of preparedness, uncertainty and lack of open dialogue. The two conditions of Becoming Menopausal are Exploring Meaning and Living with Symptoms.

Exploring Meaning. Women perceived menopause as something older women go through and chronological age did not influence response, that is, women closer to the natural menopause age of 51 years did not appear more ready or accepting. The meaning of menopause for these women was equated with feeling old.

I have to say that it is more of a mental old, because when you are in menopause, you are supposed to be old. So, I try not to go there because I can make myself feel very old quickly, my bones are getting thinner...

The abrupt onset of amenorrhea shocked many women despite that they were told that their menses would stop because of the chemotherapy.

I had chemo, I had a period, still not believing (that they would stop) and then that was it. Nothing, no more, no spotting, no nothing, wiped out totally.

After the first round of treatment, I had one period and that was it. I've never had another one since. Never any sign of one, just absent.

Drug-induced menopause was also perceived as a non-natural body experience, which was not age appropriate.

I'd still rather get my period because of the estrogen and that's what I am supposed to be doing at my age. People older than me are having babies, so I'm suppose to be getting my period at my age...I think when you start messing around with what is supposed to happen naturally in your body, that is not a good thing. Obviously I didn't have a choice but it is not something I am thrilled about.

Infertility was not a significant issue for the women in this study. Of those who were married, decisions about having children or more children had been made prior to the diagnosis. Of the four women who were single, one had a child and none of the others planned to have children prior to the diagnosis. There were some reflections of sadness, however, related to the lost ability or choice of having children now.

Living With Symptoms. The absence or presence of symptoms defined menopause and created meaning of the experience for the individual woman.

Although some women had no symptoms other than a change in menses, hot flashes, vaginal dryness, alterations in mood, cognitive changes, weight gain and changes in libido represented commonly experienced symptoms for others (Knobf, 2001). Women's responses to symptoms ranged from accepting, being resigned and tolerating them to adjusting and taking action toward symptom relief. Responses were influenced by the uncertainty of cause (chemotherapy, breast cancer, menopause), time since treatment, level of discomfort and interference with daily activities. Early during therapy, women tried to ignore symptoms or continued on despite them. Because of this, many women learned to accommodate or "put up with" the symptoms. This reflected an adjustment to living with them, with or without making changes in their daily life. "As time went on, I got a lot of hot flashes. I eventually learned to get into them and wait them out and they would go away."

Taking action in response to symptoms included self care approaches or following recommendations from other women or healthcare providers. Women who actively searched for symptom relief measures were those who generally experienced more severe physical symptom distress. With estrogen being a relative contraindication in women with a history of breast cancer and yet, the common biomedical approach to treatment of menopausal symptoms, these women learned to live with an experience that was out of the mainstream of medical practice. This further contributed to the uncertainty and vulnerability related to the women's physical and psychological integrity.

Balancing

Vulnerability remained the basic problem for breast cancer survivors. The final stage of Balancing describes the perceived vulnerability associated with risk of cancer recurrence, risk of any other serious health condition and the strong emphasis women placed on healthy lifestyle behaviors. Three strategies (Being Wary, Keeping Healthy, and Struggling with the System) were identified, aimed at protecting the woman's physical and psychological self.

Women want to protect themselves from cancer but also protect themselves from any significant threat to their health, such as heart disease, as illustrated by one woman:

> The bigger issues for me to think about were the consequences of early menopause, osteoporosis and heart disease. The Tamoxifen was very comforting for many reasons—you are still taking a drug that is going to prevent the disease from coming back—it was like a security blanket. It was also consoling to know that it worked in terms of preventing osteoporosis and heart disease. I would just as soon be on it, to be honest. I know that there are long term side effects so probably better not to take it if you don't need it, but it was comforting.

Being Wary. This strategy reflects the responsibility that women assumed for their health. It was a conscious process that reflected a heightened awareness of risks associated with anything that affects the physical body. Women critically assessed what went into their bodies and carefully weighed what is necessary, good or potentially harmful. If any degree of harm was suspected or something was valued as not essential, women often chose to live without it. Women were particularly concerned about any product that contained estrogen but were also wary of medications in general, carefully calculating the risk-benefit profile.

> I was always a good patient and if a doctor gave me a pill I would take it. Now I am much more in tune with my body and what I put into it..it's my body. I got a prescription for hot flashes (nonhormonal drug), filled the prescription but never took it...why put something into your body that I don't absolutely have to have. That is kind of my overall attitude where it once was not my attitude. I went to the gynecologist for vaginal dryness. He suggested a new product (low dose estrogen vaginal ring) and said it was safe. After I got home and read the fine print, I decided, no, the vaginal dryness is not that bad.

Keeping Healthy. Women perceived that making their bodies as healthy as possible was essential to protecting themselves from health risks. Women began to exercise, develop healthier eating habits, gathered information on health and positive lifestyle behaviors and some took vitamins and calcium supplements. Some of the women targeted their actions toward symptom relief while others directed their actions toward minimizing health risks. "I walked, I biked, it really helped my moods."

> I really need to make an effort (to lose weight) because of having gone into menopause so early at age 45. Heart and osteoporosis—my mother had both of these. I knew I had to lose weight, get back on an exercise program, which I have done.

Struggling With the System of Care. For some women, struggling with the system of care related to the specialized structure of medical care, and for other women, this represented a strategy designed to minimize any long term healthcare risks. Specialty physicians were identified as "each having their own philosophy." One woman very concerned about the late effects of menopause, especially related to a strong family history of heart disease, describes the dilemma that specialty care raises for women:

> I know that more women die of heart disease than breast cancer but he (oncologist) is not necessarily going to be focusing in on cardiovascular effects. The oncology specialist would say, "I don't want her to take estrogen because she is at too high risk to get breast cancer again." Everybody is a specialist and they deal with whatever they deal with. He was a wonderful oncologist and I hope that he did help me beat breast cancer, but I don't want to die of heart disease at age 50.

In specialty care, referral to other specialists is common practice, such as referral to gynecology for menopausal symptoms. Most of the participants were adverse to estrogen because of the relationship (actual or potential) to breast cancer and their fears of recurrence. Gynecologists often view the benefits of estrogen as outweighing the risks, and consequently women were often caught between a conflict of their beliefs, their oncologist's viewpoints and recommendations from gynecologists for symptom relief.

> I actually had some vaginal dryness and went to a gyn doctor who wanted to give me some hormonal cream. I said absolutely not because my oncologist said no hor-

mones, nothing. The gynecologist said it is just a cream. I said, excuse me but it does absorb. He said the vaginal dryness will never go away. So, you have a conflict between the gyn and the oncology doctors—that is very interesting to me.

Summary

Breast cancer and menopause represent two major life events for women and the simultaneous occurrence creates a complex experience for young midlife women. The theory of Carrying On describes women's behaviors in response to the experience of premature menopause in the context of breast cancer. In the first stage of Being Focused, the menopause experience was downstaged by the breast cancer treatment. From there, women progressed from developing an awareness of the meaning of menopause to balancing the dynamic relationship of menopause and cancer in their lives. These data enlighten our understanding about this complex phenomenon and provide direction for our clinical practice.

Discussion

The explanatory theory of Carrying On resonates a similar pattern of coping described in the recovery of women with breast cancer (LaTour, 1996) and similar to the process of adapting to the menopause transition (McElmurrey & Huddleston, 1991; Quinn, 1991). It is a process over time that incorporates acclimation, learning and adjustment to a new physiologic and psychologic place in women's lives. There are many similar concepts in the process of adapting to breast cancer and menopause and the present study provides the integration and understanding to what has been described as separate events for women.

Related to coping with illness, including breast cancer, Morse & Penrod (1999) identified the linkages among four behavioral concepts: endurance, uncertainty, suffering and hope. Each concept is associated with a level of knowing and the authors identify both linear and nonlinear, cyclical relationships among the concepts. The concepts of endurance and uncertainty have a close conceptual relationship to the first two stages in the process of Carrying On. Endurance is defined as a present-oriented state describing how a person "gets through" with little or no room for emotional responses. There is some knowledge but not full comprehension of the situation and the focus is on making it through and maintaining control. Women in the present study were totally focused on doing and getting through the experience. The second concept, uncertainty, represents a situation becoming more comprehensible but not yet with a full understanding, leaving the patient no choice but to tolerate the present. In the present study, the lack of preparedness of women for the menopausal experience and unpredictable menopausal symptoms contributed to women's level of uncertainty. Dealing with uncertainty is a major theme for breast cancer survivors (Pelusi, 1997) that has been associated with physical symptoms, emotional distress, and fear of recurrence (Mast, 1998). And, it has further been reported that the presence of physically distressful symptoms negatively impacts quality of life and challenges the recovery process (Ganz, et al, 1998; Ferrell, Grant, Otis-Greene, Garcia, 1997; Ferrell, Grant, Funk, Otis-Green, Garcia, 1998).

Uncertainty has been reported to similarly permeate the anticipated or actual menopause experience. In a sample of women from 35 to 55 years of age, menopause was perceived as a normal developmental process, but uncertainty of what to expect from the experience was more common than positive or negative expectations (Woods & Mitchell, 1999). In natural menopause, especially in the per-imenopausal phase, physical vulnerability is associated with the unpredictable and uncertain nature of symptoms, which influences how women manage and adjust to the experience (Dickson, 1994; McElmurrey & Huddleston, 1991; Quinn, 1991).

Women who experience little or no symptom distress or who are satisfied with interventions for symptom relief are less vulnerable and generally transition through menopause uneventfully (Barbach, 1994). In contrast, when the symptom experience is not well defined, the course is unpredictable and the level of symptom distress is greater, women perceive less control and greater uncertainty about what is happening to them (Kaufert & Gilbert, 1986; Rietz, 1991). In the present study, women who experienced greater symptom distress and who were less well prepared struggled more in dealing with experience than others (Knobf, 1999).

Although the context of cancer and the artificial induction of menopause is unique to breast cancer survivors, the woman's response to aging and readiness for menopause may be similar to women who experience a natural menopause transition. Aging is embedded in the menopause process (Voda, 1997), women often do not reflect on aging until menopausal symptoms appear (Choi, 1995; Wood, 1991) and some may resent menopause coming too soon, despite its biological accuracy (Greer, 1992).

Despite similarities to women's experience in the natural menopause transition, cancer changes a person. Gloria Steinum's essay on aging (1995) describes her defiance of aging, but she goes on to describe her experience of breast cancer, illustrating how cancer takes precedence, how it transforms the way women think about their bodies, how they view life and what they do to protect themselves to enhance the quality and quantity of their lives. The present study explains women's behaviors through a lens of vulnerability from cancer and through a lens which accommodates a young midlife woman who is also menopausal.

Accepted for publication April 23, 2001.

The author thanks Cheryl T. Beck, RN, DNSc, Professor, University of Connecticut School of Nursing, and Kathy Knafl, PhD, Professor, Yale University School of Nursing, for their review and critique of the manuscript, and special gratitude extended to Renee Fox, PhD, Emeritus Annenberg Professor of Social Sciences, University of Pennsylvania and Ruth McCorkle, PhD, RN, Professor, Yale University School of Nursing, for their unconditional support and mentoring.

This study was supported by NRSA T32NR07036 (University of Pennsylvania), American Cancer Society Doctoral Scholarship, Oncology Nursing Foundation Research Grant.

Corresponding author: M. Tish Knobf, PhD, RN, FAAN, 100 Church St. South, New Haven, CT 06536-0740.

M. Tish Knobf, PhD, RN, FAAN, is Associate Professor and American Cancer Society Professor, Oncology Nursing, Yale University School of Nursing.

References

Barbach, L. (1994). The pause. New York: Signet Books.

Benoliel, J. Q. (1996). Grounded theory and nursing knowledge. *Qualitative Health Research, 6*(3), 406–428.

Chenitz, W. C., & Swanson, J. M. (1986). *From practice to grounded theory.* Menlo Park: Addison-Wesley.

Choi, M. W. (1995). The menopausal transition. *Holistic Nursing Practice, 9*(3), 53–62.

Coyne, I. T. (1997). Sampling in qualitative research. Purposeful and theoretical sampling: merging or clear boundaries? *Journal Advanced Nursing, 26,* 623–630.

Dickson, G. (1994). Fifty-something: a phenomenological study of the experience of menopause. In P. Munhill (Ed). In *Women's experience.* (pp. 117–158) New York: National League of Nursing Press.

Early Breast Cancer Trialist's Group. (1998). Polychemotherapy for early breast cancer: an overview of randomized trials. *Lancet, 352,* 930–942.

Ferrell, B. R., Grant, M., Funk, B., Otis-Green, S., & Garcia, N. (1998). Quality of life in breast cancer. Part II. Psychological and spiritual well-being. *Cancer Nursing, 21*(1), 1–9.

Ferrell, B. R., Grant, M., Otis-Greene, S., & Garcia, N. (1997). Quality of life in breast cancer Part 1: Physical and social well being. *Cancer Nursing, 20*(6), 398–408.

Ganz, P. A., Rowland, J. H., Desmond, K., Meyerowitz, B. E., Wyatt, G. E. (1998). Life after breast cancer: understanding women's health-related quality of life and sexual functioning. *Journal Clinical Oncology, 16*(2), 501–514.

Glaser, B. G. (1978). *Theoretical sensitivity.* Mill Valley: The Sociology Press.

Glaser, B. G. (1990). *Basics of grounded theory analysis. Emergence versus forcing.* Mill Valley, CA: Sociology Press.

Glaser, B. G., & Strauss, A. L. (1967). *The discovery of grounded theory: Strategies for qualitative research.* New York: Aldine De Gruyter.

Greenlee, R. T., Hill-Harmon, M., Murray, T., & Thun, M. (2001). Cancer statistics 2001. *Ca-A Journal Clinicians, 51,* 15–36.

Greer, G. (1992). *The change.* New York: Knopf.

Hutchinson, S. A. (1993). *Grounded theory: The method.* In P. L. Munhall & C. O. Boyd (Eds.), Nursing research. A qualitative perspective, (pp. 180–212). New York: National League for Nursing Press.

Kaufert, P. A. & Gilbert, P. (1986). Women, menopause and medicalization. *Culture, Medicine & Psychiatry, 10,* 7–21.

Knobf, M. T. (1990). Symptoms and rehabilitation needs of patients with early stage breast cancer during primary therapy. *Cancer, 66,* 1392–1401.

Knobf, M. T. (1998). Natural menopause and ovarian toxicity associated with breast cancer. *Oncology Nursing Forum, 25,* 1519–1530.

Knobf, M. T. (1999). The influence of symptom distress and preparation on responses of women with early-stage breast cancer to induced menopause. *Psychooncology, 8,* (6 suppl.), 88.

Knobf, M. T. (2001). The menopausal symptom experience in young midlife women with breast cancer. *Cancer Nursing, 24*(3), 201–210.

Larson, P., Carrieri-Kohlman, V., Dodd, M. J., Douglas, M., Faucett, J., Froelicher, E. S., Gorntner, S., Halliburton, P., Janson, S., Lee, K. A., Miaskowski, C., Savedra, M. C., Stotts, N. A., Taylor, D., & Underwood, P. R. (1994). A model for symptom management. *Image: A Journal Nursing Scholarship, 26*(4), 272–276.

LaTour, K. (1996). The breast cancer journey and emotional resolution: A perspective from those who have been there. In K. H. Dow (Ed), *Contemporary issues in breast cancer.* (pp. 131–142). Boston: Jones & Bartlett.

Lin, E., Aiken, J. & Good, B. (1999). Premature menopause after cancer treatment. *Cancer Practice, 7,* 114–121.

Lincoln, Y. & Guba, E. (1985). *Naturalistic inquiry.* Beverly Hills, CA: Sage.

Mansfield, P. K., & Voda, A. M. (1993). From Edith Bunker to the 6:00 news: how and what midlife women learn about menopause. *Women & Therapy, 14*(1–2), 87–104.

Mast, M. E. (1998). Survivors of breast cancer: illness uncertainty, positive reappraisal and emotional distress. *Oncology Nursing Forum, 25*(3), 555–562.

McElmurrey, B. J., & Huddleston, D. S. (1991). *Perimenopausal women: using women's stories as a theoretical underpinning for women's health.* In: D. L. Taylor & N. F. Woods (Eds.). Menstruation, Health and Illness. (pp. 213–222). New York: Hemisphere Publishing.

Morse, J., & Penrod, J. (1999). Linking concepts of endurance, uncertainty, suffering and hope. *Image: Journal Nursing Scholarship, 31,* 145–150.

Munhall, P. L. (1989). Philosophical ponderings on qualitative research methods in nursing. *Nursing Science Quarterly,* 220–228.

Munhall, P. L. & Boyd, C. O. (1993). *Nursing research: A qualitative perspective.* New York: National League for Nursing Press.

Pelusi, J. (1997). The lived experience of surviving breast cancer. *Oncology Nursing Forum, 24*(8), 1343–1353.

Quinn, A. A. (1991). A theoretical model of the perimenopausal process. *Journal of Nurse-Midwifery, 36,* 25–29.

Reitz, R. (1991). *Forward.* In D. Taylor & A. C. Sumrall (Eds), Women of the 14th Moon. Writings on Menopause. Freedom, CA: The Crossing Press.

Rodgers, B. L. & Cowles, K. V. (1993). The qualitative research audit trail: a complex collection of documentation. *Research in Nursing & Health, 16,* 219–226.

Sandelowski, M. (1995). Sample size in qualitative research. *Research in Nursing and Health, 18,* 179–183.

Schag, A. C., Ganz, P. A., Polinsky, M. L., Fred, C. Hirji, K., & Peterson, L. (1993). Characteristics of women at risk for psychosocial distress in the year after breast cancer. *Journal Clinical Oncology, 11,* 783–793.

Seibold, C., Richards, L., & Simon, D. (1994). Feminist method and qualitative research about midlife. *Journal of Advanced Nursing, 19,* 394–402.

Steinum, G. (1991). *Age-and a blessing.* In: L. Taestzsch (Ed), Hot flashes: Women writers on the change of life. (pp. 145–150). Boston: Faber & Faber.

Stern, P. N., Allen, L. M., & Moxley, P. A. (1984). Qualitative research: the nurse as grounded theorist. *Health Care for Women International, 5,* 371–385.

Strauss, A., & Corbin, J. (1990). *Basics of qualitative research.* Newbury Park: Sage.

Streubert, H. J. & Carpenter, D. R. (1995). *Qualitative research in nursing.* Philadelphia: J.B. Lippincott.

Voda, A. M. (1997). *Menopause, me and you.* The sound of women pausing. New York: Harrington Park Press.

Voda, A. M. & George, T. (1986). *Menopause.* In H. H. Werley, J. J. Fitzpatrick, & R. L. Taunton (Eds), Annual review of nursing research (pp. 57–75). New York: Springer-Verlag.

Weber, G. (1994). *Celebrating women, aging and cultural diversity.* Ontario: Arthur Press.

Wood, C. E. (1991). *A split atom.* In D. Taylor & A. C. Sumrall (Eds.), Women of the 14th moon: Writings on menopause. (pp. 193–196). Freedom, CA: The Crossing Press.

Woods, N. F. & Mitchell, E. (1999). Anticipating menopause: observations from the Seattle midlife women's health study. *Menopause, 6,* 167–173.

Young-McGaughan, S. (1996). Sexual functioning in women with breast cancer after treatment with adjuvant therapy. *Cancer Nursing, 19,* 308–319.

APPENDIX

Answers to Selected Study Guide Exercises

■ *Chapter 1*

A. 1. 1. a 2. b 3. c 4. c 5. b 6. a 7. c 8. a 9. c 10. d

A. 2. 1. a 2. b 3. d 4. a 5. b 6. a 7. b 8. d 9. b 10. c 11. a 12. a

B. 1. Florence Nightingale 2. Nursing education 3. Clinical practice
4. Tradition 5. Inductive 6. Scientific method 7. Naturalistic 8. Logical positivism (positivism) 9. Empirical 10.Determinism 11. Generalizability
12. Reductionist 13. Field 14. Quantitative research 15. Qualitative research
16.Identification

C. 5 a. Basic b. Applied c. Applied d. Basic e. Basic f. Basic
g. Applied

■ *Chapter 2*

A. 1 1.a 2. c 3. b 4. a 5. b 6. a 7. c 8. c 9. c 10. b 11. a 12. a

A. 2 1. a 2. c (e.g., in milligrams) 3. d 4. b 5. a 6. a 7. c 8. d 9. a
10. c 11. a 12. b

A. 3 1. b 2. c 3. b 4. a 5. b 6. c 7. c 8. c

B. 1. Principal investigator (project director) 2. Subjects, study participants
3. Concepts 4. Variable 5. Categorical 6. Continuous 7. Independent
8. Dependent 9. Independent 10. Extraneous 11. Data 12. Operational definitions 13. Qualitative 14. Patterns of association 15. Cause-and-effect
(causal) 16. Functional (associative) 17. Reliability, validity
18. Trustworthiness 19. Triangulation 20. Bias 21. Independent variable,
dependent variable 22. Generalizability, transferability

C. 3 *Independent:* a. Participation or nonparticipation in assertiveness training
b. Patients' postural positioning c. Amount of touch by nursing staff

d. Frequency of turning patients   e. History of abuse during childhood   f. Patients' age and gender   g. Number of prenatal visits   h. Children's experience of a sibling death   i. Gender   j. Method of preoperative teaching
k. Participation in a support group   l. Time of day   m. Congruity of nurses' and patients' cultural backgrounds   n. Educational attainment   o. Setting of childbirth: home versus hospital

Dependent: a. Nursing effectiveness   b. Respiratory function   c. Patients' psychological well-being   d. Incidence of decubitus   e. Abusive behavior toward own children   f. Tolerance for pain   g. Labor and delivery outcomes
h. Depression   i. Compliance with a medical regimen   j. Anxiety levels of patients   k. Coping   l. Hearing acuity among the elderly   m. Patient satisfaction with nursing care   n. Frequency of breast self-examination   o. Parents' satisfaction with childbirth experience

■ *Chapter 3*

A.   1   1. a   2. b   3. a   4. c   5. c   6. a   7. b   8. c   9. d   10. c   11. b   12. a

A.   2   1. c   2. b   3. a   4. a   5. b   6. d   7. e   8. b   9. c   10. d

B.   1. Qualitative, quantitative   2. Intervention (treatment)   3. Grounded theory, phenomenology, ethnography   4. Phenomenology   5. Grounded theory
6. Quantitative   7. Hypotheses   8. Clinical fieldwork   9. Research design
10. Population   11. Sample   12. Empirical (data collection)   13. Data analysis
14. Pilot study   15. Research report, journal article   16. Dissemination
17. Gaining entrée   18. Gatekeepers   19. Emergent   20. Saturation

C.   2   a. In a nonexperimental study, there would not be an "active" variable.
b. The independent variable is relaxation therapy (the intervention) and the dependent variable is pain.   c. Extraneous variables are not controlled in grounded theory studies.   d. Study participants would not be randomly selected in phenomenological studies.   e. In experimental studies, decisions about data collection would be made in advance.

C.   4   a. Ethnographic   b. Phenomenological   c. Grounded theory

■ *Chapter 4*

A.   1   1. b   2. c   3. a   4. b   5. a   6. c   7. b   8. a

A.   2   1. a   2. c   3. d   4. a   5. b   6. d   7. a   8. c   9. b   10. d   11. b   12. c
13. b   14. a   15. c

B.   1. Research problem   2. Research question   3. Research aims, objectives
4. Experience, literature, social issues, theory, external sources   5. Qualitative

6. Unfeasible   7. Unresearchable   8. Feasibility   9. Relationship   10. Two
11. Independent, dependent   12. Multivariate, complex   13. Null (statistical)
14. Directional, deduction

C.   7   Independent: 5a. Type of stimulation (tactile versus verbal)
5b. Nurses versus patients   5c. Primary versus team nursing   5d. Frequency of
turning patients   5e. Patients' gender   6a. Prior blood donation versus no prior
donation   6b. Frequency of initiating conversation   6c. Nurses' informativeness
6d. Draining versus no draining of peritoneum   6e. Method of delivery

Dependent: 5a. Physiologic arousal   5b. Perceived importance of physical versus emotional needs   5c. Patient satisfaction   5d. Incidence of decubitus ulcers
5e. Amount of narcotic analgesics administered   6a. Amount of stress
6b. Patients' ratings of nursing effectiveness   6c. Level of preoperative stress
6d. Incidence of infection   6e. Incidence of postpartum depression

■ *Chapter 5*

A.   1   1. c   2. d   3. b   4. a   5. c   6. e   7. d   8. b   9. c   10. e

A.   2   1. d   2. a, b   3. a, b, c   4. a   5. b   6. d   7. a   8. a   9. b, c   10. b, c

B.   1. Research ideas   2. Findings from previous studies   3. Primary
4. CINAHL   5. Subject   6. Textword   7. Indexes, abstract journals   8. Journal
articles   9. Introduction, method section, results section, discussion
10. Relevance   11. Quotes   12. Gaps   13. Critical summary   14. Tentativeness

■ *Chapter 6*

A.   1   1. c   2. e   3. d   4. e   5. d   6. a   7. b   8. d

A.   2   1. c   2. d   3. f   4. a   5. e   6. b

B.   1. Invented (created, constructed)   2. Hypotheses   3. Framework
4. Conceptual models   5. Words   6. Probability   7. Weights   8. Person, environment, health, nursing   9. Induction   10. Health Belief Model   11. Borrowed
theories   12. Grounded

■ *Chapter 7*

A.   1. d   2. b   3. c   4. b   5. a   6. d   7. b   8. a   9. c   10. a   11. b   12. d

B.   1. Dilemmas   2. Nuremberg code   3. *Belmont Report*   4. Harm
5. Minimal risks   6. Self-determination   7. Full disclosure   8. Anonymity
9. Vulnerable   10. Institutional Review Boards

■ Chapter 8

A. 1   1. d   2. a   3. b   4. a   5. c   6. d   7. a   8. b   9. c   10. a

A. 2   1. c   2. b   3. a   4. b   5. c   6. a   7. d   8. b

A. 3   1. b   2. b   3. a   4. d   5. b   6. a   7. d   8. a   9. b   10. d

B.   1. Experimental, nonexperimental   2. Comparison   3. Flexible (unstructured)   4. Cross-sectional   5. Follow-up studies   6. Independent   7. Treatment (intervention)   8. Systematic bias   9. Random assignment   10. Factorial design continuation   11. Table of random numbers   12. Pretest (baseline measure)   13. Double blind   14. Levels   15. Crossover   16. Causality (causal relationships)   17. Comparison   18. Preexperimental   19. Time series   20. Equal (equivalent)   21. Nonexperimental   22. Correlational   23. Causation   24. Retrospective   25. Case-control   26. Incidence   27. Preceded (came before)   28. Relative risk

C.   6   a. Cannot   b. Can   c. Can   d. Cannot   e. Cannot   f. Cannot   g. Can   h. Cannot   i. Can   j. Can   k. Cannot   l. Can   m. Can   n. Cannot

C.   7   5a. Both   5b. Nonexperimental   5c. Both   5d. Both   5e. Nonexperimental   6a. Nonexperimental   6b. Both   6c. Nonexperimental   6d. Both   6e. Nonexperimental

■ Chapter 9

A.   1. a   2. a   3. c   4. b   5. c   6. a   7. b   8. b   9. c   10. a

B.   1. Constancy   2. Counterbalancing   3. Generalizability   4. Independent   5. Matching (pair matching)   6. Balanced   7. Analysis of covariance   8. Pretest (preintervention, baseline)   9. Statistical conclusion   10. Precision   11. Powe   12. On-protocol analysis   13. Internal   14. Mortality   15. Maturation   16. History   17. Target   18. External

■ Chapter 10

A.   1. a, b, c, e   2. b   3. e   4. d   5. c   6. a   7. b   8. a-f   9. a   10. f

B.   1. Randomized clinical trials (RCTs)   2. Preference   3. Beneficiaries   4. Process (implementation) 5. Net impacts   6. Cost-benefit, cost-effectiveness   7. Intervention theory   8. Outcomes research   9. Structure, process, outcomes   10. Identical (literal), virtual (operational)   11. Methods   12. Telephone   13. Census   14. Mixed-mode   15. Key informant   16. Unit of analysis   17. Meta-analysis   18. Panel of experts

■ *Chapter 11*

A. 1. b   2. a   3. d   4. c   5. b   6. a   7. b   8. c   9. d   10. c

B. . 1. Emergent   2. Bricoleurs   3. Anthropology, psychology, sociology
4. Cultures   5. Macroethnography, microethnography   6. Researcher as instrument   7. Essence   8. Spatiality, corporeality, temporality, relationality
9. Reflexive journal   10. Hermeneutics   11. Grounded theory   12. Constant
comparison   13. Formal grounded theory   14. Historical research
15. Secondary   16. Findings aids   17. Case studies   18. Narrative
19. Qualitative outcome analysis   20. Metasynthesis   21. Critical theory
22. Participatory action research

C.   2   a. Grounded theory   b. Ethnography   c. Discourse analysis
d. Phenomenology

■ *Chapter 12*

A. 1. c   2. a   3. b   4. d   5. a   6. c   7. b   8. c   9. c   10. a

B. 1. Complementary   2. Qualitative, quantitative   3. Incremental   4. Validity
5. Instruments   6. Interpretation   7. Two-stage   8. Black box   9. Epistemologic
10. Costly (expensive)   11. Component   12. Integrated

■ *Chapter 13*

A. 1   1. c   2. a   3. d   4. b   5. d   6. b   7. c   8. d   9. a   10. d

A. 2   1. b   2. c   3. a   4. b   5. b   6. c   7. a   8. a   9. d   10. b

B. 1. Sample   2. Representativeness   3. Biased   4. Homogeneous
5. Judgmental sample   6. Strata   7. Accidental, volunteer   8. Simple random
9. Sampling frame   10. Weighting   11. Multistage   12. Sampling interval
13. Sampling error   14. Accessible   15. Increases   16. 30   17. Information
18. Homogeneous, maximum variation   19. Typical case   20. Theoretical
21. Confirming, disconfirming   22. Key informants

C.   4   a. Cluster (multistage)   b. Convenience   c. Systematic   d. Quota
e. Simple random

■ *Chapter 14*

A. 1. a   2. a, b   3. b, c   4. c   5. b   6. b   7. a-c   8. a, b   9. a-c   10. a-c

B. 1. Structure, quantifiability, researcher obtrusiveness, objectivity
2. Researcher obtrusiveness   3. Biophysiologic measures   4. Self-report
5. Observation   6. Qualitizing   7. Data needs (types of data needed)
8. Subgroup effects   9. Manipulation check   10. Conceptual appropriateness
11. Readability   12. Permission   13. Pretested   14. Protocols   15. Computer-
assisted personal interviews (CAPI)   16. Ethnography   17. Audiotaped, transcribed   18. Going native

■ *Chapter 15*

A. 1   1. b   2. a   3. c   4. a   5. d   6. a   7. a   8. b   9. d   10. c   11. c   12. b

A. 2   1. c   2. c   3. a   4. c   5. d   6. a   7. d   8. b   9. c   10. c

B. 1. Grand tour   2. Descriptive, structural, contrast   3. Topic guide   4. Focus
group interview   5. Life histories   6. Critical incidents   7. Think-aloud
8. Closed-ended (fixed-alternative)   9. Open-ended   10. Closed-ended (fixed-
alternative)   11. Questionnaire   12. Dichotomous   13. Matrix questions
14. Declarative   15. Undecided (uncertain)   16. Reversed   17. Semantic differential (SD)   18. Neutral (nondirective)   19. Interview   20. Random
21. Extreme response set   22. Exclusive

C. 6   Score of Y = 11; score of Z = 26

C. 7   A = acquiescence; B = none; C = extreme response set; D = naysayers
bias

C. 8   Maximum score = 50 points; minimum score = 10 points: a. 5   b. 1
c. 1   d. 5   e. 5   f. 1   g. 5   h. 5   i. 5   j. 1

■ *Chapter 16*

A. 1. c   2. b   3. a   4. a   5. c   6. b   7. b   8. a   9. b   10. a

B. 1. Behaviors, characteristics   2. Molecular   3. Concealed   4. Intervention
5. Participant observation   6. Reflective observations   7. Selective   8. Single,
multiple, mobile   9. Log (field diary)   10. Theoretical, methodologic, personal
11. Category system   12. Molecular   13. Sign system   14. Time sampling
15. Trained   16. Error of leniency   17. Central tendency   18. Error of severity

■ *Chapter 17*

A.   1. e   2. a, c, f   3. a, c, e   4. e   5. b   6. b-e   7. b, c, e   8. f   9. g   10. d
11. b, c   12. a

B.   1. In vivo   2. Instrumentation system   3. In vitro   4. Economic   5. Middle
(center)   6. Response-set bias   7. Ipsative   8. Pictorial   9. Association
10. Vignettes

■ *Chapter 18*

A.   1   1. a   2. c   3. b   4. c   5. a   6. d   7. b   8. d   9. a   10. b

A.   2   1. a   2. c   3. b   4. d   5. a   6. b

B   1. Attributes (characteristics)   2. Quantification   3. Rules   4. True score
5. Measurement error   6. True score   7. Stability   8. Correlation coefficient
9. Positive   10. Perfect   11. Negative (inverse)   12. Homogeneity
13. Interrater (interobserver) reliability   14. Valid   15. Face   16. Content
17. Predictive   18. Convergence   19. Discriminability   20. Sensitivity, specificity
21. Efficient   22. Precision   23. Credibility, transferability, dependability, confirmability   24. Prolonged engagement   25. Data triangulation   26. Member
checking   27. Confirmability   28. Inquiry audit

C.   2   a. .77   b. 15   c. .88

■ *Chapter 19*

A.   1   1. d   2. a   3. d   4. a   5. c   6. a   7. b   8. d   9. c   10. b   11. b   12. a

A.   2   1. b   2. a   3. c   4. d   5. d   6. b   7. b   8. a   9. c   10. a

B.   1. Classification (categorization)   2. Ordinal   3. Zero   4. Equal distances
5. Statistic, parameter   6. Inferential statistics   7. Frequency distribution
8. Sample size (number of cases)   9. Frequency polygons   10. Symmetric
11. Negatively   12. Unimodal   13. Normal distribution (bell-shaped curve)
14. Central tendency   15. Mean   16. Mode   17. Variability (dispersion)
18. Homogeneous   19. Semiquartile range   20. Deviation score   21. Variance
22. Bivariate statistics   23. Cross-tabulation   24. Scatter plot   25. Pearson's *r*
(product-moment correlation coefficient)

C.   2   a. Interval   b. Ordinal   c. Ratio   d. Ratio   e. Nominal   f. Ratio
g. Interval   h. Nominal   i. Interval   j. Ratio

C. 3 Unimodal, fairly symmetric

C. 4 Mean = 81.8; median = 83; mode = 84

C. 5 a. 45 b. 3 c. 27.8% d. 2.2% e. 66.7%

C. 6 a. Sum of b. Mean c. Frequency d. Number of cases e. Raw score
f. Deviation score g. Standard deviation

C. 8 $r = -.03$

■ *Chapter 20*

A. 1. b 2. a 3. d 4. b 5. c 6. a 7. a 8. b 9. d 10. a 11. d 12. a
13. a 14. b

B. 1. Normal 2. Sample size 3. Population mean 4. Type I
5. Parametric 6. Nonparametric 7. Levels of significance 8. Type II
9. Median 10. *F* ratio 11. Mean square 12. Interaction 13. Kruskal-Wallis
14. Expected frequencies 15. Chi-square test 16. Ordinal 17. Repeated-
measures ANOVA 18. Phi coefficient 19. Nonsignificant (not statistically significant) 20. Effect size

C. 4 a. Chi-square test, Fisher's exact test, or the phi coefficient b. *t*-Test for
independent samples c. Pearson's *r* d. Median test, Mann-Whitney *U* test, or
Cramér's *V*

C. 5 a. 958 b. .113 c. Yes d. $p = .002$ (2 in 1000) e. Depression, physical health, and mental health scale scores f. The correlation between the two
variables (-.643) indicates a fairly strong and statistically significant relationship
between the two variables. Respondents who had high depression scale scores
tended to have low mental health scores (i.e., the scale is a measure of *positive*
mental health).

■ *Chapter 21*

A. 1. a, b, d 2. a-e 3. a 4. c 5. d, e 6. b 7. a-e 8. c 9. b 10. a, b, e

B. 1. Regression coefficient, intercept constant 2. Residuals 3. *R* 4. Multiple
correlation 5. Stepwise 6. Standard scores 7. Beta weights 8. Analysis of
covariance 9. Covariate 10. Multiple classification analysis 11. Factors
12. Factor extraction, factor rotation 13. Eigenvalues 14. Orthogonal,
oblique 15. Discriminant analysis 16. Canonical correlation 17. Multivariate
analysis of variance 18. Path diagram 19. Exogenous 20. Recursive
21. Maximum likelihood 22. Life table (survival) 23. LISREL 24. Latent

C.   4   a. Discriminant analysis (or logistic regression)   b. ANCOVA   c. MANO-VA   d. Multiple regression

■ *Chapter 22*

A.   1. a   2. e   3. d   4. c (also d)   5. b   6. a (also e)   7. d   8. a   9. e   10. b

B.   1. Numeric   2. Nominal   3. Quantitative   4. Precategorized (precoded)
5. Collectively exhaustive   6. Missing values   7. Identification number (ID)
8. Verification   9. Cleaned   10. Documented   11. Missing values (missing data)
12. Bias   13. Rectangular matrix   14. Transformed   15. Item reversal
16. Pooled   17. Table shells   18. Results   19. Accuracy   20. Power analysis
21. Test statistics, probability levels   22. Hypotheses   23. Generalizability
24. Correlation   25. Retained, rejected

■ *Chapter 23*

A.   1. a-c   2. a   3. b   4. a-c   5. a   6. c   7. d   8. c   9. a, b   10. d

B.   1. Simultaneously   2. Comprehending, synthesizing, theorizing, recontextual-izing   3. Indexing, categorizing   4. Conceptual file   5. Computerized methods
6. Themes   7. Constant comparison   8. Open coding   9. Selective   10. Basic
social process   11. Emergent fit   12. Strauss and Corbin   13. Phenomenological
14. Detailed   15. Domain, taxonomic, componential, theme   16. Quasi-statistics

■ *Chapter 24*

A.   1. a   2. b   3. d   4. a   5. b   6. c   7. a   8. d   9. c   10. b

B.   1. Poster session   2. Manuscript   3. Lead author   4. IMRAD
5. Introduction   6. Method   7. Results   8. Tables   9. Figures   10. Discussion
11. Journal articles   12. Alphabetically

■ *Chapter 25*

A.   1. e   2. b   3. a   4. b   5. d   6. c   7. d   8. a   9. d   10. c

B.   1. Abstract   2. Work plan   3. Budget   4. Evaluation criteria
5. Grantsmanship   6. Research Project Grant (R01)   7. Peer review (study sec-tion review)   8. Priority score   9. Pink sheets   10. Grants, contracts
11. Request for proposal   12. Request for application

C.   2   a. Research design and methods   b. Specific aims   c. Preliminary studies
d. Research design and methods   e. Human subjects (or Research design and
methods)   f. Background and significance

■ *Chapter 26*

A.   1. b   2. c   3. b   4. d   5. c   6. a   7. d   8. c   9. a   10. a   11. c   12. d
13. c   14. d   15. a

B.   1. Decisions   2. Strengths, weaknesses (limitations, flaws)
3. Substantive/theoretical   4. Methodologic   5. Ethical   6. Interpretive
7. Stylistic/presentational

■ *Chapter 27*

A.   1. c (also d)   2. a   3. a, b   4. d   5. a   6. a (also b, c, and d)   7. c (also a,
b, and d)   8. d   9. b, d   10. c

B.   1. Research utilization   2. Gap   3. Rogers' Diffusion of Innovations Theory
4. Conduct and Utilization of Research in Nursing (CURN)   5. Research utilization, evidence-based practice   6. Cochrane   7. Evidence hierarchy   8. Meta-
analyses of RCTs   9. Stetler   10. Knowledge-focused, problem-focused
11. Integrative review   12. Implementation potential   13. Ancestry, descendancy
14. Sensitivity   15. Fail-safe